Low Carb

The proven Formula To Lose Weight with Low Carb, High Fat Diet

(Simple High Protein Low Carb Recipes)

Francis Sherman

Published by Jason Thawne Publishing House

© Francis Sherman

Low Carb: The proven Formula To Lose Weight with Low Carb, High Fat Diet

(Simple High Protein Low Carb Recipes)

All Rights Reserved

ISBN 978-1-989749-26-5

This document is geared towards providing exact and reliable information in regards to the topic and issue covered. The publication is sold with the idea that the publisher isn't required to render accounting, officially permitted, or otherwise, qualified services. If advice is necessary, legal or even professional, a practiced individual in the profession should be ordered.

- From a Declaration of Principles which was accepted and approved equally by a Committee of the American Bar Association and a Committee of Publishers and Associations.

In no way is it legal to reproduce, duplicate, or even transmit any part of this document in either electronic means or in printed format. Recording of this publication is strictly prohibited and any storage of this document isn't allowed unless with proper written permission from the publisher. All rights reserved.

The information provided herein is stated to be truthful and consistent, in that any liability, in terms of inattention or otherwise, by any usage or abuse of any policies, processes, or directions contained within is the solitary and also utter responsibility of the recipient reader. Under no circumstances will any legal responsibility or blame be held against the publisher for any reparation, damages, or monetary loss due to the information herein, either directly or indirectly.

Respective authors own all copyrights not held by the publisher.

The information herein is offered for just informational purposes solely, and is universal as so. The presentation of the information is without contract or any type of guarantee assurance.

The trademarks that are used are without any consent, and also the publication of the trademark is without permission or backing by the trademark owner. All trademarks and brands within this book are for clarifying purposes only and are the owned by the owners themselves, not affiliated with this document.

TABLE OF CONTENTS

Part 1 1

Introduction 1

Chapter 1: Low Carb Diet: What It Is All About........... 3

Chapter 2: How Following A Low Carb Diet Affects Your Body And Mind................................... 5

Chapter 3: Basic Principles Of A Low Carb Diet..........14

Chapter 4: What To Eat And What To Avoid 19

Chapter 5: One-Week Sample Meal Plan 22

Chapter 6: Breakfast Recipes 26

1. BLACK BEAN, MUSHROOM AND AVOCADO BREAKFAST SCRAMBLE 26
2. BLUEBERRY POPOVERS WITH BERRY SALAD...................27
3. FRITTATA FLORENTINE 29
4. FRESH FRUIT MUESLI 30
5. ONION & CHIVE CAULIFLOWER HASH BROWNS 33
6. BRAIN BOOSTING SMOOTHIE 35
7. CHOCOLATE CHERRY SMOOTHIE 36
8. ANTIOXIDANT WAKE UP SMOOTHIE 36
9. CRUNCHY NUT COLESLAW..37
10. CREAM OF SPINACH SOUP..39
11. POACHED SALMON STEAKS WITH HORSERADISH AND CHIVE SAUCE..40

12. Lebanese Chicken Thighs..42
13. Snappy Rice Dish 44
14. Tomato-Roasted Mackerel 45
15. Cheesy Cauliflower Breadsticks 46
16. Keema Curry With Cucumber Raita 48
17. Fish With Spicy Green Lentils.................................50

Chapter 8: Dessert Recipes 54

18. Chocolate Pudding With Raspberries 54

Conclusion 55

Part 2 58

Introduction..59

1. Peaches & Cream Smoothie (Servings: 2).................66
2. Fruity-Tooty Smoothie (Servings: 2).......................68
3. Sweet Potato & Lentil Soup Moroccan Style (Servings: 3)..69
4. High Protein Enchilada Wraps Vegan Style (Servings: 7) 71
5. Soya & Veggie Burgers (Servings: 4) 72
6. Hearty Fruit Smoothie (Servings: 2) 75
7. Lemon & Lime Bitter Twist Smoothie 76
8. Chick Pea & Lentil Curry (Servings: 8)....................77
9. Bean Tortilla Wraps (Servings: 4 Wraps) 79
10. Quorn Chicken & Lentil Risotto (Servings: 4)........81
11. Chocolate Mousse (Servings: 2) 83
12. Quorn Sausage & Garlic Wedges (Servings: 2)......84
13. Quorn Ham, Cheese & Spring Onion Toasty Vegan Style (Servings: 2) 86
14. Chicken Quorn Curry (Servings: 4) 87

15. D.I.Y Chocolate Orange Protein Bars (Servings: 8) 89
16. Sweet Banana Soya Smoothie (Servings: 2) 91
17. Apple & Blueberry Porridge (Servings: 2)...............92
18. Banana With Passion (Servings: 2) 93
19. Whole Wheat Veggie Tortillas (Servings: 2) 94
20. Creamy Chicken Whole Wheat Wraps (Servings: 2) 96
21. Tropical Frozen Yogurt (Servings: 2) 98
22. Bed Of Salmon With Orange, Mango And Blackberry Juice (Servings: 2) 99
23. Muesli Fruit Mix (Servings: 3) 100
24. Mixed Fruit Energy Bars (Servings: 4).................102
25. Salmon, Asparagus & Sweet Potato Fries...........103
26. Vegetable Risotto (Servings: 3) 105
27. Mixed Bean Stir Fry (Servings: 3).......................107
28. Sweet Chicken Tikka Tortillas.............................109
29. Sweet Tuna Salad 111
30. Bass Fish Fillet With Fries 112
31. Turkey Burger 114
32. Mixed Beans On Toast..116
33. Hearty Breakfast..117
34. Turkey, Rice & Veg (Servings: 2)..........................118
35. Peanut Butter & Chocolate Sandwich With Banana (Servings: 2)..120
36. Bagel With A Treat...121
37. Chick Pea Salad (Servings: 2)..............................122
38. Posh Fish & Chips (Servings: 2) 124
39. Bed Of Avocado + Chocolate Milk (Servings: 2)..126
40. Sweet Chicken Curry (Servings: 2) 127
41. Chicken Salad With Personality (Servings: 2)......129

42. Banana & Peanut Butter English Muffin With Sweets (Servings: 2) 131
43. Chicken Pasta With Greens (Servings: 2) 132
44. Banana & Blueberry Pancakes (Servings: 2) 134
45. Creamy Tuna Pasta (Servings: 2) 135
46. Sticky Jerk Chicken (Servings: 2) 137
47. Fruit & Berry Porridge (Servings: 2) 139
48. Egg & Bacon English Muffin 140
49. Jamaican Inspired Rice & Peas – Simmer 60 Mins (Servings: 3) 142
50. Chicken Fried Rice (Servings: 2) 144

Part 1

Introduction

"There is no such thing as an essential carbohydrate... Anyone who tells you to start eating carbohydrates in order to fix a health problem is totally missing the point" – Nora Gedgaudas, Nutritional Educator and Therapist.

For many years, we have been told that carbohydrates are the main source of energy. We've been told to pair that with a very low fat intake to help us lose weight and keep it off. The problem however is that obesity seems to be becoming a worldwide pandemic with an estimated 30 percent of the world's population being overweight or obese.

While there can be many explanations for the pandemic, many studies have been pointing the blame on carbohydrates. There is an explanation to that; excessive intake of carbohydrates has been linked to a wide array of negative effects like weight gain, increased risk of diabetes, high blood pressure among other problems. This means that if you want to lose your weight among other things, the way to go is to limit your carbohydrate intake. While you may know that you need to limit your carbohydrate intake, you may not know how to get started. This is where this book comes in.

This book will provide an in-depth look at the low carb diet, how it promotes weight loss, improve health markers on some chronic conditions and diseases such as diabetes, heart disease, high blood pressure, sleep disorders among many others. You will also learn how to get started.

Thanks again for downloading this book, I hope you enjoy it!

Chapter 1: Low Carb Diet: What It Is All About

Low Carb Diet: What Is It?

In its simplest terms, a low carb diet simply involves cutting down your carbohydrate intake while increasing consumption of foods that are high in protein and or fat.

So what exactly is considered low carb?

In general, the fewer carbs you consume, the better results you get. Even the phrase "low-carb diet" does not have a legal definition and this has resulted in many interpretations by many. This is why the amount of carbohydrates you consume depends on your dietary needs. However, according to Dr. Jennifer Fitzgibbon, an Oncology dietitian at the New York's Stony Brook Hospital Cancer Center, the phrase "low-carb diet" is essentially applicable to diets that restrict carbohydrates to just under 20% of caloric consumption. A low carb diet can also imply a diet that limits carbohydrates to less than the suggested proportions, which are usually below 45% of the total energy derived from carbohydrates.

The idea behind this is to switch the body from relying on carbohydrates for energy to fats or proteins for energy, a phenomenon that ultimately brings about weight loss and a host of other benefits. As I already stated in the introduction, it is important to reiterate that carbohydrates are not essential macronutrients as we have been made to believe for a long time. This means that you can thrive even without them since your body can obtain the energy it requires from the other two macronutrients (fats and proteins).

With that understanding of a low carb diet, let us now look at what you stand to benefit by adopting a low carb diet.

Chapter 2: How Following A Low Carb Diet Affects Your Body And Mind

In order to understand how a low carb diet works, you should first know what happens you eat a meal that is high in carbohydrates; your pancreas secretes hormone insulin, which breaks down the carbohydrates to glucose. If your meals are too high in carbohydrates, the excess glucose is converted to glycogen and stored in the liver and muscle tissues. Since the storage space for glycogen in the liver and muscles is usually limited, the liver converts the remaining glucose into fatty acids and triglyceride in a process known as lipogenesis, which has no limit to the quantity of fat it can synthesize. These fats are then transported and deposited in different organs of the body, therefore weight gain.

When you consistently reduce the amount of carbohydrates you consume, your insulin level lowers and the little glucose produced is not enough to provide enough energy to sustain the whole body. This prompts your body to turn to the liver and muscles for stored glycogen since it is easily within reach.

The glycogen is first re-converted to glucose and respiration occurs to provide an instant dose of energy for the body cells. The glycogen stores in the liver and muscle tissues are enough to provide the body with glucose for a day or a day and a half before they are completely depleted.

When glycogen is exhausted from the liver and muscle, the body reaches deeper into fat stores all around the body. It is from this point onwards that the body starts to burn fat to provide the body with energy and this will keep up as long as you are on a low carb diet.

With that explanation f how a low carb diet works, let us now look at some of the benefits you are likely to enjoy:

Weight Loss

If you are struggling to lose weight, then you will find limiting your carbohydrate intake one of the most simple and effective ways to shed those stubborn extra pounds. The great news is that you will achieve that without having to endure any hunger pangs.

As explained above, reducing your carbohydrate intake makes your body to burn fat for energy, which definitely leads to weight loss. In addition, you will not be storing any excess glucose in form of fat since your carbohydrate intake is low.

Improved Stamina (physical endurance)

A low carbohydrate diet can increase your stamina immensely because it gives you continuous access to all the energy produced when your fat stores are being used up. Your fat stores have enough energy to carry you through for a few weeks or even months. This is in contrast to when your body is relying on using glucose and stored carbohydrates (glycogen) for energy as it only lasts for a few hours.

The body usually has the capacity to store a lot of fat and the body fat content clearly dwarfs the glycogen stores that are only stored in small quantities in the liver and muscles. This means that once your body fully adapts to burning fat rather than using glycogen, you can perform for long periods in endurance events such as long distance running without having to replenish yourself with extra food for energy.

Another reason why you would want to utilize your body fat rather than carbohydrates for fuel in endurance activities is that fats are usually very energy dense. This means that they provide the most concentrated form of energy than all the other macronutrients. Fats provide more than double the amount of energy that proteins and carbohydrates do (fats contain 9 calories in every gram as compared to 4 calories per 1 gram of carbohydrates (sugars and starches) or proteins and 1.5 – 2.5 calories per every gram of fiber). This is also the reason why your body tends to use fat to store energy over a long period while using carbohydrates to store energy for the short term.

Less Appetite and Cravings

The reason why many people give up on dieting is that they cannot tolerate the severity of their hunger pangs any further. However, one of the main advantages of following a low carb diet is that it reduces your appetite and helps you beat cravings. This is because when you limit the amount of carbohydrates and sugars in your diet and include more healthy fats and proteins, you feel more satiated.

In addition, usually, high levels of insulin in the bloodstream regulate the production of ghrelin. Further, 'high density lipoproteins' are a 'carrier particle' for the efficient circulation of ghrelin. In simple terms, what this means is that when you consume carbohydrates, the level of insulin in your blood elevates to suppress the production of ghrelin and converts the carbs to blood sugar, which is used as fuel by your body. But when the blood sugar levels drop, ghrelin levels increase and this stimulates hunger and sugar cravings.

On the contrary, the consumption of fats and proteins has been shown to turn on the satiety hormone known as leptin whose function is to send signals to your brain telling it that you have eaten to your fill and therefore you should stop eating.

The only way to have your insulin levels under control is reducing your carbohydrate intake.

Reduced Blood Pressure

This study shows that a low carb diet can normalize high blood pressure. When left untreated, high blood pressure poses serious health threat such as a heart attack or a stroke. If you reduce your carb intake to less than 100 grams every day, then you can reduce blood pressure by a significant margin. But how exactly can a low carb diet lower your blood pressure?

A low carb diet can lower blood pressure by reducing the amount of intra-abdominal fat that is deposited within the abdominal cavity. This fat induces the production of a number of chemicals and hormones that lead to an increase in blood pressure and some of these are:

Leptin hormone, which is produced by the adipose tissues to regulate hunger. However, it also stimulates the SNS (sympathetic nervous system) which contributes to the vasoconstriction (constriction of the blood vessels such that they become narrower and stiffer) and ultimately high blood pressure

ROS (reactive oxygen species) which also stimulates the SNS and the ARAS (ascending reticular activation system and contributes to vasoconstriction

Increased Cortisol production, which can cause increased retention of sodium in the kidneys, which leads to vasoconstriction and eventually high blood pressure

Low adiponectin production, which leads to vasoconstriction

Moreover, a low carb diet improves insulin resistance and reduces the chances of the

SNS being activated. This dilates and relaxes the blood vessels and reverses the abnormal withholding of sodium from the kidneys.

Reversal of Type 2 Diabetes

Type 2 diabetes is a condition in which the body no longer responds adequately like it should to insulin. As a result, the body has to find a way to produce more insulin to bring down the high blood sugar levels. Scientists have hypothesized that for your body to control blood sugar levels effectively, you ought to adopt a low carb diet.

Studies show that a low carb diet is effective in preventing insulin resistance. Another study conducted by scientists from the University of Naples showed impressive results of a low carb Mediterranean diet on type 2 diabetes patients over a period of 8 years. Just 12 months into the study, 15% of the patients had already achieved remission (diabetes reversal). By the end of the sixth year 5%

more of the patients also achieved remission.

So what principles should you follow in order to be considered as following a low carb diet and be certain of positive results? That's what we will discuss next.

Chapter 3: Basic Principles Of A Low Carb Diet

The main goal of a low carb diet is to limit your carbohydrate intake while increasing your protein and fat intake. The good news is that you can limit your carbohydrate intake and decide either to increase your protein intake or fat intake or even both.

Let us look at the different types of low carb diet so that you can choose one that is best suited for your needs.

The Ketogenic Diet

This is an incredibly low carb and high fat diet. It comprises of a carb percentage of 5% or below. This amounts to between 20 and 50 grams of net carbohydrates per day. The protein and fat content should be 20% and 75% respectively.

The aim of the keto diet is to maintain carb consumption at the lowest point possible to allow the body to switch to a metabolic state known as ketosis. Ketosis is a process in which the liver breaks down fat through oxidation to form ketones (energy molecules) such as acetoacetate and beta-hydroxybutyrate (BHB). The ketones produced are an alternative source of energy when glucose is absent.

When you are on the ketogenic diet, your body switches almost entirely to run on ketones produced from fat. Since the body organs and in particular, the brain requires a lot of energy to function; the diet should include plenty of fats.

Atkins Diet

Like any other low carb diet, this diet was developed to promote weight loss and improve health markers among overweight patients. It was named after Dr. Robert C. Atkins who published a book about this diet in 1972 and it went on to receive worldwide plaudit.

Health experts and Dietitians who advocate for this diet believe that you can get rid of body fat by consuming as much fats and proteins as you need, provided that you do away with foods that are high in carbs.

The Atkins diet has been split into 4 distinct phases. The first (induction) phase that should last for 2 weeks requires that you consume less than 20 grams of carbs every day, which corresponds to 10% of the daily calorie intake while eating high protein and high fat foods and this is considered the recipe that initiates weight loss. Proteins should take up 20%-30% of the daily calorie intake while fats should take up 60%-70%. On the balancing phase, which is the 2nd phase, you can include some low carb veggies, more nuts and fruits. Continue with the balancing phase then switch gears to the fine-tuning phase when you get closer to your weight goal. On the last (maintenance) phase, you can eat as many healthy carbs as you please but be careful not to overdo this to prevent regaining back the lost weight.

South Beach Diet

Dr. Arthur Agatston, a Florida-based cardiologist, developed this diet in the

1990's. He observed how the Atkins diet produced impressive weight loss results on overweight people. However, he was against the idea of eating plenty of saturated fats in the Atkins diet especially for people with heart complications. He was also against the idea of limiting foods such as whole grains and fruits, which are high in fiber and have 'good carbs'.

This prompted him to slightly modify the Atkins Diet to come up with the South Beach diet, which is low in glycemic index carbs but higher in lean proteins and healthy unsaturated fats. The macronutrient ratio remained the same as that of the Atkins diet. He believed this diet would not only help diabetic or overweight patients to lose weight, but it would also reduce their risk of developing heart disease.

The South Beach diet is divided into three phases. Phase one is usually considered to be very strict, lasts for two weeks and is designed to do away with cravings, normalize blood sugar levels and initiate weight loss. You should eat three meals per day that are composed of unsaturated fats, proteins and non-starchy vegetables/fruits. You should stay in phase two for as long as possible until you reach your desired weight. During this phase, consume all foods from phase 1 but restrict the portions of fruit and 'good carbs' like grains. Once you achieve your weight goal, move on to phase three observe the guidelines in phases 1 and 2 but you can allow occasional treats but do not overindulge to avoid gaining the weight you lost.

In the following chapter, we will look at the foods you can eat and those to avoid irrespective of the type of low carb diet you decide to adopt.

Chapter 4: What To Eat And What To Avoid

Avoid The Following Foods And Drinks:

All sugars and sweet foods – candy and sweets, sweeteners, pastries, buns cakes, chocolate, ice cream, juices, soda, sports drinks, breakfast cereals

All processed foods – Eat real food rather than packaged sugar free and low carb processed foods that still contain lots of preservatives, fillers and other harmful ingredients.

Beer – usually made from barley and is high in carbs

Fruits – contain a lot of sugar; thus, should be eaten occasionally.

Starchy foods - Breads and pasta (foods made from wheat, rye, barley, spelt etc), rice, porridge, muesli, potatoes, French fries, potato chips, Legumes such as lentils and all beans, moderate consumption of root vegetables such as carrots.

N.B: Many companies are shamelessly tricking their consumers into believing that their products are 'low carb' yet they are producing processed foods with high amounts of sugars, sugar alcohols, salt, flour and toxic additives. It is up to you to avoid all these processed foods at all costs.

Foods To Eat:

Meat and poultry – beef, game, pork, lamb, chicken, veal, turkey; the fattier the better

Fish and other seafood – shellfish, salmon, cod, mackerel, trout, tuna, shrimp, haddock, sardines, herring etc

Organic eggs

Fats and oils – butter or ghee, palm, coconut, hemp, olive, flaxseed, walnut and lard oils

Vegetables – especially the ones grown above the ground e.g. broccoli, mushrooms, cauliflower, spinach, kale, cabbage, cucumber, zucchini, peppers, chard

Dairy produce – opt for full fat products e.g. cheese, sour cream, real butter, Greek yogurt. Limit regular milk, low fat and skimmed milk and avoid sweet flavored products

Drinks – water, unsweetened green, black, white and oolong teas, herbal teas, coffee, green smoothies, fresh pressed vegetable juices.

Let's put all the above into perspective by discussing a meal plan that will ensure you succeed in your quest to switching to a low carbohydrate way of life.

Chapter 5: One-Week Sample Meal Plan

Monday

Breakfast	Scrambled eggs with a serving of vegetables fried in either coconut oil or butter
Lunch	Shrimp salad dressed in olive oil
Dinner	Baked salmon with butter and lemon

Tuesday

Breakfast	Bacon and eggs
Lunch	Previous night's leftovers
Dinner	Cheeseburger (without buns) with salsa and vegetables

Wednesday

Breakfast	Bacon, Spinach and Cheese Frittata

Lunch	Previous night's leftovers
Dinner	Grilled chicken with vegetables

Thursday

Breakfast	Omelet with vegetables fried in either coconut oil or butter
Lunch	Meat pie with vegetables
Dinner	Pork chops with steamed broccoli

Friday

Breakfast	Green Smoothie
Lunch	Garlic chicken with vegetables fried in

	butter
Dinner	Pork chops with blue cheese sauce

Saturday

Breakfast	Almond Pancakes with blueberries
Lunch	Chicken breast with herb butter
Dinner	Bacon wrapped meatloaf

Sunday

Breakfast	Mushroom omelet
Lunch	Hamburger patties

	with creamy tomato sauce
Dinner	Salmon tandoori with cucumber sauce

Chapter 6: Breakfast Recipes

1. Black Bean, Mushroom and Avocado Breakfast Scramble

Serves: 2
Ingredients:
- 4 teaspoons oil
- 2 cups white button mushrooms, sliced
- 4 large eggs, whisked
- Freshly ground pepper to taste
- Salt to taste
- 1 small avocado, peeled, pitted, diced
- ½ cup onion, diced
- 2 small cloves garlic, finely minced
- ½ cup canned or cooked black beans, rinsed
- 2 tablespoons fresh cilantro, chopped (optional)

Method:
1. Place a skillet over medium heat. Add oil. When the oil is heated, add onions and mushrooms and sauté until soft.

2. Add garlic and sauté until fragrant. Add beans, salt and pepper. Pour eggs over it. Keep stirring until the eggs are set.
3. Divide into 2 plates. Place avocado slices on top. Garnish with cilantro and serve.

2. Blueberry Popovers with Berry Salad

Serves: 4

Ingredients:

<u>For blueberry popovers:</u>

- ½ cup all-purpose flour
- ½ teaspoon stevia
- ½ cup 1%coconut milk
- ½ tablespoon stevia
- A pinch salt
- 1 egg
- ¼ cup blueberries
- Cooking spray

<u>For berry salad:</u>

- ½ cup raspberries
- ½ cup strawberries, hulled, cut into thick slices
- ½ cup blueberries
- 1 teaspoon sugar

Method:

1. To make blueberry popovers: Grease 4 muffin cups with cooking spray and set aside.
2. Add flour, salt and sugar into a bowl. Make a cavity in the mixture and crack the egg into it. Add milk and beat using a wire whisk until smooth.
3. Pour the batter into the prepared muffin cups. Fill up to 2/3. Sprinkle a few blueberries is each.
4. Bake in a preheated oven at 425ºF for 25 -30 minutes or until golden brown on top.
5. Meanwhile make the berry salad as follows: Blend most of the raspberries and pass through a wire mesh strainer. Discard the seeds. Add the puree into a bowl.
6. Add rest of the ingredients into the bowl and mix well.

7. When the popovers are ready, allow it to cool for 5 minutes. Run a knife around the edges of the popovers and remove it carefully.
8. Sprinkle icing sugar on it.
9. Serve warm with salad.

3. Frittata Florentine

Serves: 2

Ingredients:
- 2 tablespoons red onion
- 2 teaspoons extra virgin olive oil
- ½ cup spinach or arugula, chopped
- ¼ cup canned sweet corn
- 2-3 tablespoons parmesan cheese, grated (optional)
- 1 clove garlic, minced
- 1 plum tomato, chopped
- ½ red bell pepper, chopped
- 4 eggs, beaten
- Salt to taste
- Pepper to taste

Method:
1. Place an ovenproof skillet over medium heat. Add oil. When the oil is heated, add onion and garlic and sauté until translucent.
2. Add tomatoes, spinach, corn and bell pepper. Cook for 2-3 minutes.
3. Whisk together eggs, salt and pepper into a bowl and pour over the vegetables in the skillet. Cook until the sides begin to set. Remove from heat.
4. Sprinkle cheese on it.
5. Transfer the skillet into a preheated oven.
6. Bake at 350ºF for 25 -30 minutes or until cheese melts and the eggs are set in the center.

4. Fresh Fruit Muesli
Serves: 3

Ingredients:
- ¼ cup bulgur
- 1 tablespoon sunflower kernels
- 1 green apple, cored, grated
- ½ passion fruit
- ¼ cup pomegranate seeds or blueberries to garnish
- 6 tablespoons rolled oats
- ¼ cup almonds, slivered
- 1 peach or nectarine, pitted, chopped + extra to garnish
- ½ teaspoon pure almond extract

Method:
1. Soak bulgur in a bowl of water. Cover and set aside for 30 minutes. Drain and place it in a large bowl.
2. Pass the pulp of the passion fruit through a wire mesh strainer. Press the pulp well with the back of a spoon. Add the strained juice into the bowl of bulgur.
3. Add rest of the ingredients and fold gently.
4. Cover and chill until use.

5. Garnish with blueberries and peach and serve.

5. **Onion & Chive Cauliflower Hash Browns**

Serves: 4

Ingredients:

- 4 cups cauliflower, grated to get rice like texture
- Salt to taste
- 1 small onion, finely chopped
- 1 tablespoon red bell pepper, finely chopped
- 1 tablespoons green bell pepper, finely chopped
- Freshly ground pepper to taste
- 4 teaspoons olive oil
- 2 small blocks onion and chive Cotswold cheese, grated
- 2 large eggs

Method:

1. Add cauliflower, salt, pepper, eggs, green bell pepper and red bell pepper into a bowl and mix well.

2. Place a nonstick pan over medium high heat. Add olive oil and swirl the pan. When the oil is heated, spoon about ¼ the mixture on the pan and flatten it with the back of a spoon or a spatula.
3. Cook until the underside is golden brown. Flip sides and cook the other side.
4. Sprinkle cheese over it when you flip sides.
5. Repeat with the remaining mixture to make 3 more.
6. Serve hot.

6. Brain Boosting Smoothie

Serves: 2

Ingredients:

- 2 handfuls hemp nuts
- 2 teaspoons Rhodiola rosea
- ½ cup blueberries
- 1 cup apple juice
- Ice cubes as required

Method:

1. Add all the ingredients to a blender and blend until smooth.
2. Pour into tall glasses and serve.

7. Chocolate Cherry Smoothie

Serves: 2-3

Ingredients:

- 2 cups spinach
- 2 cups frozen cherries
- 1 teaspoon ground cinnamon
- 2 cups almond milk, unsweetened
- 3 teaspoons cacao powder

Method:

1. Add all the ingredients to a blender and blend until smooth.
2. Pour into tall glasses and serve.

8. Antioxidant Wake up Smoothie

Serves: 2

Ingredients:

- ½ cup blueberries
- 1 ½ cups vanilla almond milk
- 1 cup frozen cherries
- 1 ½ teaspoons green tea powder
- Stevia (optional)

Method:
1. Add all the ingredients to a blender and blend until smooth.
2. Pour into tall glasses and serve.

Chapter 7: Lunch / Dinner Recipes

9. Crunchy Nut Coleslaw

Serves: 2

Ingredients:
- 3.5 ounces white cabbage, finely shredded
- 2 ½ tablespoons sultanas
- 1 tablespoon low fat mayonnaise
- Pepper to taste

- 3 tablespoons peanuts, roasted
- 1 small radish, thinly sliced
- 1 medium carrot, grated
- 2 green onions, finely chopped (both the whites and greens)
- 5 tablespoons high fat yogurt
- 2 tablespoons fresh parsley, chopped to garnish

Method:
1. Mix together mayonnaise, yogurt and pepper in a bowl.
2. Add rest of the ingredients into the bowl and mix until the vegetables are well coated.
3. Garnish with parsley and serve immediately.

10. Cream of Spinach Soup

Serves: 3

Ingredients:

- 1 medium red onion, chopped into chunks
- ½ tablespoon tamari sauce
- 2 ½ cups water
- 2 teaspoons chicken soup powder
- 2 cups fresh spinach
- 1 tablespoon coconut oil
- ½ cup (38% fat) whipping cream

Method:

1. Place a skillet over medium heat. Add oil. When the oil is melted, add onions and sauté until translucent.
2. Add spinach and tamari and sauté until the spinach wilts. Add water and bring to the boil.
3. Add soup powder and stir constantly until it is well combined. Let it simmer for 5 minutes.

4. Remove from heat. Blend with an immersion blender until smooth.
5. Place the skillet back on low heat. Add cream and stir. When it is heated (do not boil), remove from heat.
6. Ladle into soup bowls and serve.

11. Poached Salmon Steaks with Horseradish and Chive Sauce

Serves: 2

Ingredients:
- 1 cup 2% coconut milk
- 1 tablespoon lemon juice
- 1 stalk celery with leaves, chopped
- 2 black peppercorns
- 2 teaspoons bottled grated horseradish
- ¼ cup high fat mayonnaise
- Freshly ground pepper to taste
- ¾ cup water
- 2 tablespoons onion, thinly sliced
- 1 small carrot, chopped
- 2 salmon steaks (4 ounces each)

- ¼ cup high fat sour cream
- 1 tablespoon fresh chives, chopped

Method:
1. Place a nonstick pan over medium heat. Add milk, water, onion, celery, carrots and peppercorns and bring to the boil.
2. Lower heat and simmer for 7-8 minutes. Add salmon and lemon juice and stir. Cover with a lid.
3. Cook until the fish flakes easily when pierced with a fork. Remove from heat.
4. Remove the salmon with a slotted spoon and place on a plate lined with paper towels. Discard the liquid in the pan.
5. Meanwhile mix together sour cream, horseradish, chives, mayonnaise and pepper in a bowl. Set aside.
6. Place the salmon on 2 serving plates. Divide the horseradish mixture and place over the salmon.
7. Serve immediately.

12. Lebanese Chicken Thighs

Serves: 4

Ingredients:

- 4 tablespoons ghee
- 4 Roma tomatoes, halved
- 8 chicken thighs
- 10-12 baby carrots
- 30 cloves garlic
- Juice of 2 lemons
- Garlic olive oil as required
- Pepper to taste
- Salt to taste
- 2 Vidalia onion, quartered
- 2 teaspoons dried oregano

Method:

1. Grease a large cast iron pan with about 3-4 teaspoons garlic olive oil.
2. Place the chicken thighs on it. Do not overlap the chicken. Leave a little space in between 2 chicken thighs.

3. Place onions, carrots, garlic and tomatoes in between the chicken thighs. Place a few garlic cloves on top of the thighs.
4. Sprinkle lemon juice over the chicken. Sprinkle some more garlic oil over the chicken. Pour melted ghee over it.
5. Sprinkle salt, pepper and oregano.
6. Bake in a preheated oven at 500°F for about 30 minutes.
7. Lower the temperature and bake at 350°F for 20 minutes or the internal temperature of the chicken is 165°F.
8. Broil for a few minutes and cook until crisp.
9. Serve hot.

13. Snappy Rice Dish

Serves: 4

Ingredients:
- 2 cups vegetables, fresh or frozen, cut into bite size pieces
- 2 cups cauliflower, grated to a rice like texture
- 2 tablespoons fresh dill or 2 teaspoons dried dill
- 1 cup broth or water
- 14 ounces chickpeas or kidney beans or pink beans
- Pepper to taste

Method:
1. Add vegetables and broth into a saucepan and place over medium high heat. Cook until tender.
2. Add rest of the ingredients and heat thoroughly.
3. Serve hot.

14. Tomato-Roasted Mackerel

Serves: 2

Ingredients:

- ½ pound mackerel fillets
- 2 tablespoons fresh basil leaves, chopped
- ¼ teaspoon salt
- 2 tablespoons low fat mayonnaise
- 1 large tomato, sliced
- Pepper to taste

Method:
1. Place mackerel on a lined baking sheet. Spread 1-tablespoon mayonnaise on each.
2. Place tomato slices and basil on top. Season with salt and pepper.
3. Bake in a preheated oven at 400°F for about 5-10 minutes or until mackerel turns opaque.

15. Cheesy Cauliflower Breadsticks

Serves: 4

Ingredients:

- 2 cups cauliflower, grated to a rice like texture
- 1 cup mozzarella cheese, shredded + extra to top
- 2 teaspoons, garlic, minced
- ½ teaspoon red pepper flakes or to taste
- Pepper to taste
- 1 ½ teaspoons dried oregano
- Salt to taste
- 2 eggs, beaten

Method:

1. Line a baking dish with parchment paper. Set aside.
2. Add cauliflower rice to a microwave safe bowl and cover. Microwave on high for 8-10 minutes.
3. Transfer into a bowl. Add garlic flakes and red pepper flakes and mix well. Add salt and oregano. Mix well.
4. Add eggs and mozzarella cheese. Mix well.
5. Transfer the mixture into the prepared baking dish. Press well.
6. Bake in a preheated oven at 350°F for 30 minutes.
7. Remove from oven. Sprinkle some more mozzarella cheese.
8. Bake for another 8-10 minutes or until the cheese melts.
9. Remove from oven and slice.
10. Serve hot.

16. Keema Curry with Cucumber Raita

Serves: 2

Ingredients:

- 1 pound lean ground beef
- 1 cm fresh ginger, finely chopped
- ½ teaspoon turmeric powder
- ½ teaspoon coriander seeds, crushed
- 9 ounces canned diced tomatoes with its juice
- Pepper to taste
- Salt to taste
- 1 medium onion, finely chopped
- 1 cup baby spinach
- 2 cloves garlic, chopped

- 1 inch stick cinnamon
- ½ teaspoon cumin seeds, crushed
- ¼ teaspoon crushed dried chili
- ¾ cup low salt beef stock
- Fresh mint leaves to garnish

For cucumber raita:

- ½ cup plain, high fat yogurt
- 2 teaspoons fresh mint, chopped
- 2 tablespoons cucumber, finely chopped
- Pepper to taste

Method:

1. Place a skillet over medium heat. Add beef and sauté until brown. Break it simultaneously as it cooks.
2. Add the garlic, ginger, chili, cumin, coriander, cinnamon stick, crushed red chill and pepper and sauté for a couple of minutes. Stir constantly.

3. Add tomatoes and stock and bring to the boil.

4. Cover with a lid and simmer until potatoes and meat are cooked.

5. Add spinach and heat until it wilts. Taste and adjust the seasonings if necessary. Remove from heat.

6. Meanwhile, make cucumber raita as follows: Add all the ingredients of cucumber raita in a bowl. Mix well and refrigerate until use.

7. To serve: Ladle curry into bowls. Garnish with mint leaves and serve with cucumber raita.

17. Fish with Spicy Green Lentils

Serves: 2

Ingredients:

- 1 tablespoon extra virgin olive oil
- 1 stalk celery, chopped
- 1 large mild red chili, deseeded, finely chopped
- 1 ½ cups low salt vegetable stalk
- 1 small bay leaf
- A pinch cayenne pepper
- 2 white fish fillets (5 ounces each), skinless
- Pepper to taste
- 1 small onion, chopped
- 1 leek, chopped
- 6 ounces dark green lentils, rinsed, drained
- 1 sprig fresh thyme
- Juice of ½ lemon
- Lemon wedges to serve

Method:

1. Place a skillet over medium heat. Add ½ tablespoon oil. When the oil is heated, add onion, celery, chili and leek and sauté for a couple of minutes.

2. Add stock, lentils, thyme and bay leaf and bring to the boil.

3. Reduce heat and cover with a lid. Simmer until tender. If there is liquid remaining in the skillet, then drain the excess liquid.

4. Place fish in a broiler pan with the skin side facing up.

5. Mix together in a bowl, ½ tablespoon oil, and cayenne pepper and lemon juice and brush this mixture over the fish.

6. Sprinkle salt and pepper over it.

7. Broil in a preheated oven until the fish flakes when pierced with a fork.

8. To serve: Divide the lentils in 2 serving dishes. Place the fish on top and serve garnished with lemon wedges.

53

Chapter 8: Dessert Recipes

18. Chocolate Pudding with Raspberries

Serves: 4

Ingredients:

- 8 ounces chocolate(85%) pudding
- 2 cups raspberries
- 4 tablespoons whipped cream

Method:

1. Spoon chocolate pudding into 4 bowls. Top with raspberries and whipped cream.
2. Chill and serve.

Conclusion

We have come to the end of the book. Thank you for reading and congratulations for reading until the end.

I hope this book was able to help you to learn about the low carb diet and how you can actually adopt this diet.

The next step is to get started now and enjoy the many benefits this diet has to offer.

When you are going low-carb, you don't have to stop eating. You will simply need to cut out all carbs from your daily diet. That's about it. That does sound simple, doesn't it? Who said that dieting has got to be difficult? You might be wondering how spaghetti Bolognese would taste without any spaghetti in it? Since you are going low-carb, you will need to come up with alternatives for all the carbs you are used to eating. Zucchini noodles could be substituted for pasta. Well, it is quite easy.

The recipes that have been given in this book are easy to follow. You can cook delicious and healthy food by following the simple steps given. The next time you have your friends and family over for a meal, you can cook them a feast by following these recipes. All that you will need to do is stock up on all the necessary ingredients you need for cooking.

Thank you and good luck!

Part 2

Introduction

You may think that a low carbohydrate and fat diet is the way forward to achieve weight loss and a healthy lifestyle but this isn't necessarily the case. The main macronutrients in the foods we consume are made up of protein, carbohydrates and fat, but it's what type and how much of each that you consume that really makes the difference. Proteins are mainly found in animal sources and by products but it's important to choose from lean sources. Lean sources of protein can be found in tuna, salmon, chicken, turkey and eggs. They can also be found in lesser amounts within nuts, legumes, beans and plant based sources. It's often thought within the fitness community, that the more protein you consume the bigger and leaner your muscles will become – but this couldn't be further from the truth. For instance, research has found that eating any more than 30g protein per meal sitting, it's not likely that your body will utilize it and therefore the excess that you can't digest will store as unused energy in the form of fat. The same can be said about carbohydrates and fats but it's going to depend on your size and genetics to be specific. Protein is essential for muscle growth and certainly contributes to you becoming leaner as it gives you that satiated feeling of fullness. Plus, as you can only consume around 20-30g protein per meal sitting, to get the sufficient amount for your body type it's a good idea to eat several small meals throughout the day. This will also help to boost your metabolism and keep your energy levels high throughout the day.

Carbohydrates are tricky, it's really important that you educate yourself on this because when you think of losing weight, people tend to cut out carbohydrates all together and this is dangerous because carbohydrates are our main energy source. Sugar or the more technical term 'glucose' is our main energy source which is released into the bloodstream to use as energy. Carbohydrates are stored in the form of glycogen within your muscles and liver and depending on the type of carbohydrate you consume determines how fast energy is released and broken down into the form of glucose. Now that you understand that not all carbohydrates are the same, it's wise that you learn to separate the good from the bad and when it's ideal to utilize both types.

There are two types of carbohydrates – 'simple' and 'complex.' Simple carbohydrates are mainly made up of fast release sugars, therefore they will convert to glucose very quickly and if the energy isn't utilized it'll be stored as fat. They are mainly found in white starchy foods such as white potatoes, white pasta, spaghetti, white rice and white bread. You may find that you can eat a lot of simple carbohydrates and this is due to how quickly they are digested and released as energy. The problem is, if you don't exercise prior to eating simple carbohydrates, long term it can really contribute to weight gain. You may agree that it takes quite a lot of simple carbohydrates to make you feel full, this is due to the fast digestion process and it's also why many people who consume excess simple sugars on a daily basis are at a high risk of developing diabetes.

Although simple carbohydrates aren't recommended to lose weight and increase your energy levels, they can be utilized very well immediately after exercise and up to two hours after. This is for recovery and to help grow and repair muscle tissue and cells and to replenish muscle glycogen stored as energy. This is why it's so important to load up on complex carbohydrates 1-2 hours before exercise, so that your muscles and liver have sufficient energy stores to fuel your workout. Hence, this is why a diet consisting of predominantly simple carbohydrates will not benefit your energy levels or workout, because of how fast the glycogen stores are converted to glucose and released into the bloodstream as unused energy. If you have no glycogen stored, then you aren't going to have sufficient energy stores to help you burn off the excess fat you're carrying. The easiest way to judge complex carbohydrates from the simple ones, is to remember that the simple carbs are mainly white and complex carbs are generally brown. Complex carbohydrates are mainly made up of wholegrains, whole wheat, wholemeal and consist of a lot of fibre which takes a long time to digest. Therefore, the process of when the glycogen is broken down, will take longer to convert to glucose and release into the bloodstream to use as energy. This is why it's best to consume mainly complex carbs if you're looking to increase your energy levels and lose weight because they will keep you fuller for longer and stop you from indulging in unhealthy foods. Fibre is released slowly, it's good for your gut and best of all it helps to release energy slowly, so by consuming a diet made up of mainly complex carbohydrates you're sure to get a steady release of energy throughout the day. Complex carbohydrates can be found in whole wheat pasta, wholegrain rice, wholemeal bread, sweet potatoes and even beans and legumes.

Just as important as carbohydrates are fats, fats are essential to us and we need them for several reasons. A small amount of unsaturated fats, are vital for your health as they help your body to absorb fat soluble vitamins such as vitamin A, D, E and they can only be absorbed with the help of other fats. We also use fat as an energy source, but it's important to note that your body will always look to use carbohydrates as its main energy source first and when the glycogen stores become depleted the body will start to utilize fat for energy. If you're a weight lifter or bodybuilder, then your main source of energy would come from carbohydrates, keep in mind that most sessions usually last around 60 minutes. Now if you look at somebody that's a long-distance endurance runner, they'll be exercising for 1-3 hours so what happens is, their body uses the glycogen stores first and as time goes on it will start to utilize fat stores.

It isn't recommended to exercise on an empty stomach because your body won't run on fat stores, it doesn't work that way, your body will begin to break down muscle tissue to utilize energy and this brings about severe fatigue. The type of fats you need to avoid are saturated fats. Too much saturated fat can contribute to high cholesterol which increases the risk of heart disease, stroke and cardiovascular disease. Its recommended that you take in no more than 30g saturated fat per day. Saturated fats are found predominantly in animal meats, butter, lard, cream, meat (sausages, bacon), chocolate and biscuits. When you look at how much of each of the macronutrients you should consume within your diet per meal, the eat well plate recommends to consume 50% Carbohydrates, 35% Protein and 15% Fat. This makes sense as over half of your plate should be made up of complex carbohydrates which are our main source of energy, over a quarter of the plate should be made up of protein which serves many roles including helping to make you feel full and a small amount of unsaturated fat which is essential.

1. Peaches & Cream Smoothie (servings: 2)

Ingredients:

- ½ tin of peaches
- 200ml skimmed milk
- 100ml frozen Greek yogurt
- ¼ cup cottage cheese
- ¼ cup oats
- 1 tsp lemon zest
- 2 tbsp. chia seeds

Nutritional benefits:

Greek yogurt, skimmed milk and cottage cheese contain lots of slow release protein, calcium and do wonders for the immune system. Try to make sure that the syrup that the peaches are contained in are low in sugar. Oats and chia seeds also contain a considerable amount of protein along with a high fibre content to provide slow release energy. The lemon zest adds a tangy twist to this recipe and contains some strong antioxidant properties to help boost the immune system.

Nutrition value:

Protein – 35g / 17.5g per serving

Carbohydrates – 63.7g / 31.8g per serving

Fat – 10.9g / 5.4g per serving

Total Kcals – 492.9 Kcals / 246.4 Kcals

The Recipes

2. Fruity-Tooty Smoothie (servings: 2)
Ingredients:

- 1 cup fresh pineapple
- ¼ cup blueberries
- 200ml pomegranate juice
- 150ml frozen Greek yogurt
- 2 tbsp. flax seeds

Nutritional benefits:

This smoothie serves as a great snack to boost your energy levels without raising blood sugar and is full of antioxidants that support your immune system and provides fuel for when you need it. The flax seeds provide some quality protein along with fibre and omega 3 fatty acids, the pineapple, pomegranate juice and blueberries provide a source of fibre, vitamin C, antioxidants and fructose which gives you a boost of energy without affecting glucose levels. Greek yogurt is a great source of slow release protein and contains plenty of calcium.

Nutrition value:

Protein – 16.8g / 8.4g per serving

Carbohydrates – 61.1g / 30.5g per serving

Fat – 9.8g / 4.9g per serving

Total Kcals – 399.8 Kcals / 199.9 Kcals per serving

3. Sweet Potato & Lentil Soup Moroccan Style (servings: 3)
Ingredients:

- 200g green lentils (uncooked)
- 200g garden peas
- Medium sweet potato (150g)
- ¼ cup water
- ½ white onion (finely sliced)
- 1 medium tomato (chopped)
- 2 tbsp. parsley
- 2 tbsp. tomato paste
- 2 garlic cloves (finely sliced)
- 1 tsp turmeric
- 1 tsp salt
- ½ tsp pepper
- ½ tsp red chilli powder

- 500 ml water

Preparation method:

Place the tomatoes, garlic, tomato paste, salt, pepper, onion and turmeric in a large non-stick pan with ¼ cup water and cook on a low heat for 5-7 minutes – stirring occasionally. Then add the lentils, peas and 500ml of water, mix together and leave to gently simmer on a low-medium heat for 30 mins or until the mix has a thick consistency. After 20 minutes add the parsley. When the mix has thickened add the chilli, mix and leave to stand for 2 minutes before serving. Meanwhile pre-heat your oven to 220 degrees, fork your potatoes several times and microwave on full power for 10 mins and then put in the oven for a further 20 minutes. Once your dish is ready, serve the lentil soup in a large bowl and potato on a side plate.

Nutrition value:

Protein – 26.8g / 8.9g per serving

Carbs – 80.1g / 26.7g per serving

Fat – 2.5g / 0.8g per serving

Total kcals – 450.1 kcals / 150 Kcals per serving

4. High Protein Enchilada Wraps Vegan Style (servings: 7)

Ingredients:

- 400g Chicken Quorn strips
- 100g tofu (cut into strips)
- 400g black beans (1 tin in water)
- 150g wholegrain rice
- 100g spinach (frozen)
- 100g mushrooms (sliced)
- 56g soy cheese
- 7 whole wheat tortillas
- 340g green chilli enchilada sauce (1 jar)

Preparation method:

Wash the black beans thoroughly to avoid gas. Cook all the above ingredients (apart from the enchilada sauce, soy cheese and tortillas) all according to packaging. Once everything is ready, put 7 tortillas on a large serving plate and place in microwave for 30-40 seconds on full power, then pack the tortillas and wrap on an oven tray tightly together length ways, side by side. Pour the enchilada sauce over and cover the wraps from top to bottom. Grate the soy cheese over the top and put in the oven on 190 degrees C for 20 minutes or until crisp. Serve immediately!

Nutrition value:

Protein – 132g / per serving – 18.9g

Carbs – 246.2g / per serving – 35.2g

Fat – 31.5g / per serving – 4.5g

Total kcals – 1796.4 kcals / per serving – 256.9 kcals

5. Soya & Veggie Burgers (servings: 4)
Ingredients:

- 4 whole wheat buns
- 2 tbsp. extra virgin olive oil
- 75g soya crumbs
- ¾ cups water
- 1 tbsp. red chilli powder
- 1 tbsp. sea salt
- ½ cup bread crumbs

- 5 mushrooms (sliced)
- ½ red pepper (chopped)
- ¼ cup fresh coriander leaves
- 3 jalapeno peppers (finely sliced)
- 1 cup soaked beaten rice/3 tbsp. red poha
- 1 large whole egg
- 4 tbsp. soya cream cheese
- 1 large tomato
- 4 tbsp. mustard
- 100g fresh spinach leaves

Preparation method:

Put soya crumbs in a large bowl and add the ¾ cup of water, leave to soak for 5 minutes or until all water has absorbed. Once absorbed, fork through the mix and add the bread crumbs – mix with the fork again. Then add the mushrooms, chopped peppers, coriander leaves, jalapeno peppers, beaten rice mix, salt and red chilli powder. Combine all the ingredients and mix well before adding the egg – mix well again. (use flax seeds and water to replace the egg if vegan). With the combined ingredients, make 4 burger patties and put to one side. Put your frying pan on a medium heat, add 1 tbsp. olive oil and wait for 2 minutes to heat up. Add one burger at a time, push down on the mix to ensure a flat surface – leave for 3-4 minutes or until the side has cooked, then flip and leave another 3-4 minutes. Once cooked, put the burger to one side, slice the bun in half and put them cut face down in the pan to lightly toast – 1-2 minutes. (Add another tbsp. olive oil after 2nd burger). Spread 1 tbsp. soya cream cheese on one half of the bun and 1 tbsp. mustard on the other half. Add the burger in between the slices along with 2 fresh spinach leaves and 2 slices of tomato. Heaven!!

Nutrition value

Protein – 99.7g / per serving – 24.9g

Carbs – 184.5g / per serving – 46.1g

Fat – 61.1g / per serving – 15.3g

Total kcals 1686.7 kcals / per serving – 345.2 kcals

6. Hearty Fruit Smoothie (servings: 2)

Ingredients:

- 1 cup fresh pineapple
- ¼ cup blueberries
- 200ml pomegranate juice
- 150ml frozen Soya yogurt
- 2 tbsp. flax seeds

Nutritional benefits:

This smoothie is a great snack to boost your energy levels without raising blood sugar and is full of antioxidants that support your immune system and provides fuel for when you need it. The flax seeds provide some quality protein along with fibre and omega 3 fatty acids, the pineapple, pomegranate juice and blueberries provide a source of fibre, vitamin C, antioxidants and fructose which gives you a boost of energy without affecting glucose levels. Soya yogurt is a great source of slow release protein and contains plenty of calcium.

Nutrition value:

Protein – 16.8g / 8.4g per serving

Carbohydrates – 61.1g / 30.5g per serving

Fat – 9.8g / 4.9g per serving

Total Kcals – 399.8 Kcals / 199.9 Kcals

7. Lemon & Lime Bitter Twist Smoothie
Ingredients:

- ¼ of a lemons juice
- 1 tsp lemon zest
- ¼ of a limes juice
- 1 tsp lime zest
- 250ml frozen vanilla soya yogurt
- 250ml coconut milk
- 1 tbsp. organic maple syrup
- 2 tbsp. flax seeds

Nutritional benefits:

The lemon and lime zest have strong antioxidant properties that protect your immune system and adds a sweet and bitter kick to any desert. The lemon and lime juice contain lots of vitamin C which is great for the absorption of iron, they also boost the immune system as they contain lots of antioxidant properties. Flax seeds are known as one of the top power foods as they're packed with energy dense nutrients including fibre, protein, healthy fatty acids and fibre, they can help to lower your blood pressure, reduce cholesterol and fights inflammatory. Coconut milk is lower in fat when compared to animal milk, it's full of calcium also that help to keep your bones strong. Soya yogurt is also full of calcium and has a considerable amount of slow digesting protein.

Nutrition value:

Protein – 15g

Carbohydrates – 32.9g

Fat – 19g

Total kcals – 362.6 kcals

8. Chick Pea & Lentil Curry (Servings: 8)
Ingredients:

- 2 tbsp. curry powder seasoning
- 1 tbsp. coriander seasoning

- 1 tbsp. cumin seasoning
- 1 tsp chilli powder seasoning
- 3 tbsp. extra virgin olive oil
- 3 garlic cloves (finely sliced)
- 1 medium white onion (finely sliced)
- ½ a lemons juice
- ½ a limes juice
- 100ml coconut milk
- 1 tin of organic tomatoes (400g)
- 400g tin of chick peas (in water)
- 200g green lentils (uncooked)
- 600g white rice (long grain, uncooked)
- 1 organic chicken stock cube
- 500ml water for the stock
- 1.2L water for rice

Preparation method:

Thoroughly wash the chick peas and lentils and leave to one side – preferably over a 24hour period. Heat a large pan on a low-medium heat and add the olive oil – leave for 2 minutes and then add the garlic and onion. Cook until the onion is translucent. Meanwhile dissolve 1 chicken stock cube in 500ml of boiling water. Once the onions are translucent add the lentils and fry for 1-2 minutes before adding the chicken stock and all the seasoning. Add a little bit of stock at a time just covering the lentils – keep the heat on medium – high. Once all the stock has been absorbed, add the chick peas and tin of tomatoes and allow to simmer on a low heat for 25-30 minutes stirring occasionally. For the last 20 minutes add the rice and 1.2L water to another pan and boil on a medium-high heat.

Nutrition value

Protein – 62.9g / 7.9g per serving

Carbohydrates – 334.5g / 41.8g per serving

Fat – 54.4g / 6.9g per serving

Total kcals – 2079.2 kcals / 259.9 kcals per serving

9. Bean Tortilla Wraps (servings: 4 wraps)
Ingredients:

- 200g tinned red kidney beans (in water)

- 200g tinned reduced salt and sugar baked beans
- 200g mixed beans (in water)
- X4 plain tortilla wraps
- 2 handfuls salad leaves
- 100g mixed peppers (chopped)
- 1 tbsp. garlic seasoning
- 1 tbsp. paprika seasoning

Preparation method:

Start by thoroughly washing the red kidney and mixed beans and then add to a medium sized pan along with the baked beans in tomato sauce and seasoning. Cook on a low heat and simmer for 10-12 minutes. Once the bean mix is done, throw the tortillas in the microwave on full power for 40 seconds, fill them with the bean mix, add the salad leaves and wrap. Serve with raw peppers on the side. Nutritious and delicious!!

Nutrition value

Protein – 39.9g / 10g per serving

Carbohydrates – 107.7g / 26.9g

Fat – 8.1g / 2g

Total kcals – 663.3 kcals / 165.8 kcals

10. Quorn Chicken & Lentil Risotto (Servings: 4)

Ingredients:

- 1 medium white onion
- 3 garlic cloves (finely sliced)
- 3 sprays 1 calorie pam oil
- 200g green lentils (uncooked)
- 100g Quorn chicken
- 300g Arborio risotto rice
- 2 tbsp. balsamic vinegar
- 100g vine tomatoes
- 2 pinches of sea salt & cracked black pepper for risotto
- 2 pinches of sea salt & cracked black pepper for tomatoes
- ½ courgette (chopped)
- 50g violife original vegan cheese or alternative (grated)
- 2 organic chicken stock cubes
- 1L water

- 1 sprig of fresh rosemary

Preparation method: To begin with set your oven to 180 degrees and then add in a small baking tray the tomatoes with rosemary on top, salt and pepper seasoning and drizzled balsamic vinegar over the top and cook for 30-35 minutes. Then put a large frying pan on a low-medium heat with the pam oil and leave for 2 minutes before adding the onion and garlic — cook until the onion turns translucent. Then add the Quorn chicken and cook until golden brown. While you're waiting for the Quorn to cook, prepare your chicken stock dissolving the 2 chicken stock cubes in 1L of boiling water. Once the Quorn is ready add your lentils and risotto rice and wait 2 minutes before adding the stock — add a little at a time just covering the mix. Turn the heat high and cook to the boil, then turn the heat back down again and simmer until all the stock has been absorbed. Once you are half way through the chicken stock (500ml) add the chopped courgettes and push them into the mix. Once all the water has been absorbed, the final step is to turn off the heat and add the cheese alternative and salt and pepper seasoning and leave to stand for 2 minutes. Stir the melted cheese through and then serve with the tomatoes on top. Simply irresistible.

Nutrition value:

Protein – 45.4g / 11.3g per serving

Carbohydrates – 143.4g / 35.8g per serving

Fat – 24.9g / 6.2g per serving

Total kcals – 979.3 kcals / 244.8 kcals per serving

11. Chocolate Mousse (servings: 2)
Ingredients:

- 1 scoop chocolate soya protein powder
- ¼ cup water
- ½ avocado (ripe)
- ¼ cup slithered almonds (crushed)
- ½ cup ice

- 2 tbsp. green and black's dark chocolate cocoa powder (>70% cocoa)

Preparation method:

Blend the water and protein powder together then add the chocolate powder, ¾ of the slithered almonds and avocado and blend again. If you're going to eat it straight away throw in the ice for 30 seconds, if not pour the mix into a small bowl and put into the fridge. Sprinkle the remaining crushed almonds over the top of the mousse before you eat and enjoy!

Nutrition value:

Protein – 36.3g / 18.1g per serving

Carbs – 25.6g / 12.8g per serving

Fat – 27.2g / 13.6g per serving

Total Kcals – 492.4 Kcals / 246.2 Kcals per serving

12. Quorn Sausage & Garlic Wedges (servings: 2)
Ingredients:

- 200g white potato
- 2 Quorn meat free sausages
- 150g mixed vegetables
- 1 tbsp. extra virgin olive oil
- 1 tbsp. garlic seasoning
- 1 rosemary sprig
- 1 pinch sea salt and black pepper
- Salsa (50g)

Preparation method: Pre-heat your oven to 220 degrees. Cut the potato into thick wedges, drizzle the olive oil over them and season with the rosemary, garlic, salt and pepper. Place them into the microwave on full power for 10 minutes. when done place into the oven, cook for a further 20 minutes or until crisp. For the last 15 minutes of the wedges crisping in the oven, add the Quorn sausages to the oven and cook until golden brown. For the last 10 minutes add the mixed vegetables to a small pan and boil on a high heat.

Nutrition value:

Protein – 20.8g / 10.4g per serving

Carbs – 52.4g / 26.2g per serving

Fat – 17.3g / 8.6g per serving

Total Kcals – 448.5 Kcals / 224.2 Kcals per serving

13. Quorn Ham, Cheese & Spring Onion Toasty Vegan Style (servings: 2)
Ingredients:

- 3 slices Quorn meat free ham
- 2 whole wheat slices of bread
- 30g violife original vegan cheese (or any other brand of vegan cheese)
- 3 spring onions (finely chopped)
- 2 handfuls mixed salad
- 250ml organic orange juice
- X2 sprays 1 calorie pam oil

Preparation method:

Simply place the spring onions, Quorn ham and cheese alternative between the slices of bread, spray the pam oil over the outside of both slices and put under a sandwich toasty or George Foreman grill until the bread is golden and toasted on the outside of both sides. Serve with the mixed salad on the side and with a fresh glass of orange juice.

Nutrition value:

Protein – 13.5g / 6.8g per serving

Carbs – 63.5g / 31.7g per serving

Fat – 11.7g / 5.8g per serving

Total Kcals – 413.3 Kcals / 206.6 Kcals

14. Chicken Quorn Curry (servings: 4)
Ingredients:

- 300g Palau rice (ready-made 2-minute rice)
- 200g Quorn chicken
- 150g frozen peas
- 1 chicken stock cube
- 500ml water for the stock
- 2 white medium onions (chopped)
- 3 garlic cloves (finely sliced)
- 1 heaped tbsp. flour
- 100ml coconut milk
- 2 tbsp. soya yogurt
- ½ limes juice
- ½ lemons juice

- 1 tbsp. coriander seasoning
- 1 tbsp. chilli cayenne seasoning
- 1 tbsp. garam masala seasoning
- 1 tsp salt
- 3 sprays 1 calorie pam oil spray

Preparation method:

In a large frying pan spray in the pam and leave to heat up for 2 minutes on a low-medium heat. Then add the onions and garlic – cook until the onions are translucent. Next, add the Quorn chicken and cook until golden brown, while you're waiting prepare your stock by dissolving the chicken stock cube in 500ml of boiling water. Once the chicken is ready pour in the frozen peas and begin to add the stock along with the seasoning, add the stock a little at a time just covering the mix. Once you poured in the last bit of stock, add the flour, stir and continue cooking for a further 2 minutes then add the coconut milk, lime and lemon juice and simmer on a low heat until the mix begins to thicken. Once the curry sauce is cooked to your desire, turn the heat off and add the soy yogurt, leave to stand for 2 minutes and then stir. The final step is to simply pop your Palau rice into the microwave and heat for 2 minutes.

Nutrition value:

Protein – 53.5g / 13.4g per serving

Carbohydrates – 155.7g / 38.9g per serving

Fat – 23.4g / 5.8g per servings

Total kcals – 1047.4 kcals / 261.8 kcals per serving

15. D.I.Y Chocolate Orange Protein Bars (servings: 8)
Ingredients:

- Wet mix
- ¼ cup freshly squeezed orange juice
- ¼ cup vegan dark chocolate (>70% cocoa)
- ¼ cup almond milk
- ¼ cup organic peanut butter
- ¼ cup apple sauce (unsweetened)
- ¼ cup organic maple syrup Dry mix

- 1 tbsp. orange zest
- ¼ cup raw oats
- 1 tbsp. ginger seasoning
- 3 tbsp. chia seeds
- ¼ cup slithered almonds
- ¼ cup mixed berries
- 3 scoops soya protein powder (unflavoured)

Preparation method:

Put the dry mix into a large mixing bowl and mix ingredients together. Put the wet mix in a separate bowl and put in the microwave on full power for 30 seconds or until the mix is thick and creamy. Then pour the wet mix on top of the dry mix and mix together well. Use an 8x8 container or plastic tub, put down some wax paper and spray with pam oil. Place the mix into the container and pat down until the surface is flat, then put it in the fridge for an hour to set. Cut into 8 pieces and enjoy as a desert or a snack on the go.

Nutrition value (per serving)

Protein – 17.9g

Carbohydrates – 33.8g

Fat – 19.3g

Total kcals – 380.7 kcals

16. Sweet Banana Soya Smoothie (servings: 2)

Ingredients:

- 1 large banana
- 250ml unsweetened soya milk
- Pulp of one passion fruit
- 100g Greek yogurt
- ½ tsp cinnamon

Nutritional benefits:

Bananas are jam packed with potassium which helps the circulatory system and eases muscle cramps, they're high in fibre and help regular bowel function. Soya milk is a healthy alternative to cow's milk and is packed with calcium and healthy fibre along with protein. Cinnamon also has many benefits including a high antioxidant content along with antiaging properties. Greek yogurt contains a heavy amount of calcium and slow digesting protein and passion fruit is high in iron, vitamin c, fibre, and helps to reduce cholesterol.

Nutrition value

Protein – 20.8g / 10.4g per serving

Carbohydrates – 60.3g / 30.1g per serving

Fat – 6.6g / 3.3g per serving

Total Kcals – 383.8 Kcals / 191.9 Kcals

17. Apple & Blueberry Porridge (servings: 2)

Ingredients:

- ½ cup raw oats
- 190ml skimmed milk
- 1 apple (chopped)
- ¼ cup blueberries (frozen)
- 1 tsp unsweetened apple sauce

Preparation method:

In a medium sized pan add the entire ingredients apart from the apple sauce and put on the hob on a low-medium heat for 3-4 minutes or until the porridge thickens to your desire – stirring frequently. Once the porridge has thickened to your liking, simply add the apple sauce, stir and leave to stand for 1 minute before consuming.

Nutrition value:

Protein – 12.6g / 6.3g per serving

Carbohydrates – 65.4g / 32.7g per serving

Fat – 4.8g / 2.4g per serving

Total Kcals – 355.2 Kcals / 177.6 Kcals

18. Banana with Passion (servings: 2)
Ingredients:

- 1 large banana (chopped)
- 200g natural yogurt
- Pulp of ½ a passion fruit
- 1 tsp honey

Preparation method: This is a lovely desert that can be eaten at any time of day, it's relatively low in fat, high in protein and complex carbohydrates. It's also the perfect snack before bed as bananas, Greek yogurt and honey actually promote the sleep hormone melatonin for the perfect night's sleep. In a desert bowl simply add the chopped banana, and pour the yogurt over the top along with the passion fruit pulp and drizzle the honey over the top.

Nutrition value

Protein – 10.4g / 5.2g per serving

Carbohydrates – 71.1g / 35.5g per serving

Fat – 8g / 4g per serving

Total Kcals – 398 Kcals / 199 Kcals per serving

19. Whole Wheat Veggie Tortillas (servings: 2)

Ingredients:

- 2 whole wheat tortillas
- 1 avocado (ripened)
- ½ beetroot ball (chopped into small chunks)
- 2 spring onions (finely chopped)
- 2 garlic cloves (crushed)
- 1 tbsp. olive oil
- ¼ cup white mushrooms (chopped)

- ½ red pepper (chopped)
- 1 medium carrot (grated)
- 1 small tomato (chopped into small chunks)
- 1 handful lettuce
- ¼ cup cucumber (chopped into small chunks)
- 1 tsp fresh parsley
- 1 tsp fresh oregano
- 1 tbsp. balsamic vinegar
- 1 tbsp. lime juice
- 1 pinch sea salt
- 2 tbsp. natural yogurt

Preparation method:

Add the olive oil to a large frying pan and pre-heat on a low-medium heat for 2 minutes before adding the 2 crushed garlic cloves and spring onions. Cook for 2-3 minutes and then add the chopped mushrooms, pepper, tomato along with the balsamic vinegar, lime juice and salt, oregano and parsley seasoning – cook for a further 6-7 minutes stirring frequently. Then add the natural yogurt, stir through the mix and leave to stand for 1 minute.

Next, put the tortillas in your microwave and heat on full power for 30-40 seconds, lay them out on a plate and add the mix from the pan along with the remaining ingredients; avocado, beetroot, grated carrot, lettuce and cucumber. Wrap and enjoy!

Nutrition value:

Protein – 13.3g / 6.7g per serving

Carbohydrates – 68.7g / 34.3g per serving

Fat – 19g / 9.5g per serving

Total Kcals – 499 Kcals / 249.5 Kcals

20. Creamy Chicken Whole Wheat Wraps (servings: 2)

Ingredients:

- 100g chicken fillet (skinless & chopped)
- 4 sprays 1 calorie pam oil
- 2 whole wheat tortillas
- 1 small tomato (chopped into small chunks)
- ¼ cup cucumber (chopped into small chunks)

- 1 handful baby spinach leaves
- 3 tbsp. ricotta cheese
- 1 tsp parsley
- 1 tsp fresh mint
- 1 tsp Cajun seasoning

Preparation method:

In a large frying pan add the pam oil and leave to pre-heat on the hob on a low-medium heat for 2 minutes. Meanwhile, season your chicken by rubbing the Cajun seasoning over it evenly with your hands – it's easier if you chop the chicken first. Cook the chicken for 10-12 minutes or until cooked through then add the tomato, cucumber, along with the parsley and fresh mint – cook for 3-4 minutes. Then turn the heat off, add the ricotta cheese, stir through and leave to stand for 2 minutes. While you're waiting, put the tortillas in the microwave and heat on full power for 30-40 minutes. Add the mix to the tortillas, wrap and get stuck in!

Nutrition value:

Protein – 38.8g / 19.4g per serving

Carbohydrates – 50g / 25g per serving

Fat – 12g / 6g per serving

Total Kcals – 463.2 Kcals / 231.6 Kcals

21. Tropical Frozen Yogurt (servings: 2)

Ingredients:

- 1 tbsp. crushed hazelnuts
- 1 kiwi (skinned and sliced thin)
- 1 pulp of ½ a passion fruit
- 200g Greek yogurt

Preparation method:

Another delicious recipe packed with nutrients high in healthy omega-3 fats derived from the nuts, high in protein and low in carbohydrates. Simply add the sliced kiwi and crushed hazelnuts to a desert bowl and top with the yogurt, then drizzle with the passion fruit pulp. Beautiful.

Nutrition value:

Protein – 23.8g / 11.9g per serving

Carbohydrates – 36.7g / 18.3g per serving

Fat – 28.1g / 14.1g per serving

Total Kcals – 494.9 Kcals / 247.4 Kcals per serving

22. Bed of Salmon with Orange, Mango and Blackberry Juice (servings: 2)

Ingredients:

- 1 slice smoked salmon
- 1 slice wholegrain bread (toasted)
- 1 handful baby spinach leaves
- 1 pinch sea salt and cracked black pepper

Dressing:

- 1 tbsp. light cream cheese
- 1 tsp lemon juice
- 1 tsp mustard
- 1 tsp fresh parsley

The Juice:

- 250ml 100% orange juice
- ½ medium mango (skinned and chopped)
- ½ cup blackberries
- 3 ice cubes

Preparation method:

In a small mixing bowl add the light cream cheese, lemon juice, mustard and parsley and mix together into a thick paste – leave to one side. Then, in a blender add the orange juice, blackberries and mango along with the ice cubes and blend for 1-2 minutes or until the mix is smooth – pour into a glass and put to the side. Finally, season the salmon with salt and pepper and place on top of the toasted bread along with the baby spinach leaves. Drizzle the dressing on top and serve with the juice. Delicious.

Nutrition value

Protein – 14.9g / 7.5g per serving

Carbohydrates – 67.5g / 33.7g per serving

Fat – 10.7g / 5.3g per serving

Total Kcals – 425.9 Kcals / 226.4 Kcals

23. Muesli Fruit Mix (servings: 3)
Ingredients:

- ¼ cup muesli

- ¼ cup special k
- ¼ cup blackberries
- ¼ cup strawberries
- Pulp of ½ a passion fruit
- 200g Greek yogurt
- 1 tsp honey

Preparation method:

This is one of my favourite breakfast recipes as its packed with protein and energy dense carbs in the form of fibre to help fuel your day with very little fat.

In a small glass desert bowl, add the muesli as the bottom layer, then ½ of the yogurt, then the special k, then another layer of yogurt. Top with the blackberries and strawberries and drizzle with the passion fruit pulp and honey. Warning! This will make your mouth water!

Nutrition value

Protein – 33.1g / 11g per serving

Carbohydrates – 82g / 27.3g per serving

Fat – 5.6g / 1.9g per serving

Total Kcals – 500 Kcals / 166.7 Kcals per serving

24. Mixed Fruit Energy Bars (servings: 4)
Ingredients:

- 1 handful crushed hazelnuts
- ¼ cup dates
- ¼ cup mixed dried berries
- 3 tbsp. flax seeds
- ¼ cup unsweetened apple sauce

Preparation method:

These energy bars are simple to make and full of nutrients, they taste great and can be taken with you anywhere. They mainly consist of fibre and complex carbohydrates as that is the main macronutrient that provides energy.

Start by adding the hazelnuts and flax seeds to a blender and blend for 2-3 minutes or until the mix is reasonably smooth. Then, add the rest of the ingredients and blend for a further minute. Empty the mix and add it to a medium sized plastic tub – ensure you put some wax paper inside the tub first and spray with pam oil so the mix doesn't stick. Pat the mix down so that the surface is flat and place the container in the fridge for 1 hour. Then, cut the bar into 4 servings and place back in the fridge. Eat when you're peckish or when on the go for a quick energy boost.

Nutrition value

Protein – 14.3g / 3.6g per serving

Carbohydrates – 137g / 34.3g per serving

Fat – 42.4g / 10.6g per serving

Total Kcals – 986.8 Kcals / 246.7 Kcals per serving

25. Salmon, Asparagus & Sweet Potato Fries
Ingredients:

- 100g salmon fillet
- 150g sweet potato (medium sized)
- 50g salsa
- 1 tbsp. rapeseed oil
- 4 sprays 1 calorie pam oil

- 1 tsp sea salt and black cracked pepper
- 4 sticks of asparagus
- 1 tsp garlic seasoning
- 1 tsp rosemary seasoning

Preparation method:

Pre-heat your oven to 200 degrees. Leave the skin on the potatoes and chop into 0.5 inch slices. Put them onto a plate, drizzle the rapeseed oil over them and add the garlic and rosemary seasoning – mix together with your hands. Place them into a microwave for 10 minutes on full power then add them to the oven for a further 20-25 minutes to crisp. As soon as you place the fries into the oven grab a frying pan and spray in the pam oil and leave to pre-heat for 2 minutes on the hob on a low-medium heat. Season the salmon with the salt and pepper and add to the centre of the pan – cook for 15-20 minutes, tossing occasionally. For the final 10 minutes add the asparagus to the pan. Add everything to a large serving dish along with the salsa to taste.

Nutrition value:

Protein – 29.2g

Carbohydrates – 36.5g

Fat – 22.8g

Total Kcals – 468 Kcals

26. Vegetable Risotto (servings: 3)
Ingredients:

- ½ cup risotto rice
- 1 medium white onion (diced)
- 1 cup garden peas
- ¼ cup chopped courgette
- ¼ cup carrots (chopped into small chunks)
- 30g low fat cheese (grated)
- 1 vegetable stock cube
- 600ml water
- 1 pinch sea salt and cracked black pepper
- 2 garlic cloves (crushed)
- tbsp. olive oil
- 1 tsp low fat butter

- 1 large vine tomato (chopped into quarters)
- 1 rosemary sprig
- 1 tbsp. balsamic vinegar

Preparation method:

Start by pre-heating a large wok or frying pan over a low-medium heat for 2 minutes along with the olive oil. Then, add the crushed garlic along with the diced onion and cook until the onion turns translucent. Meanwhile, heat your oven to 180 degrees and in a tray with foil add the vine tomato quarters and season with the salt and pepper, then drizzle with the balsamic vinegar along with 1 rosemary sprig – leave to roast for 30 minutes. Once the onions are ready, add the frozen peas, risotto rice, courgette and carrots and cook for 1-2 minutes while you prepare the stock. Dissolve 1 vegetable stock cube in 600ml of boiling water and add to the pan a little at a time just covering the mix. Turn the heat up high and bring to the boil, then turn the heat back down low and simmer for 25-30 minutes – stirring occasionally. Once the risotto has thickened to your desire, turn the heat off and add the butter and grated cheese – stir through and leave to stand for 2 minutes. Stir again and add the tomato mix from the oven on top, consume right away!

Nutrition value:

Protein – 25.8g / 8.6g per serving

Carbohydrates – 103.3g / 34.4g per serving

Fat – 31.3g / 10.4g per serving

Total Kcals – 798.1 Kcals / 266 Kcals per serving

27. Mixed Bean Stir Fry (servings: 3)
Ingredients:

- 1 tin mixed beans (300g in water)
- ¼ cup sweetcorn
- ½ red pepper (chopped into small chunks)
- ½ white onion (finely sliced)
- ¼ cup broccoli (chopped)

- ¼ cup carrots (grated)
- ¼ cup cucumber (chopped)
- 1 handful baby leaf spinach
- ½ medium tomato (chopped into small chunks)
- 4 sprays 1 calorie pam oil

Dressing:

- 1 tbsp. soy sauce
- 1 tsp lemon juice
- 1 tsp balsamic vinegar
- 1 tbsp. rapeseed oil
- 2 garlic cloves
- 50g salsa

Preparation method:

The first thing you need to do is to leave the beans to soak for at least an hour and then rinse thoroughly. Pre-heat your wok pan or frying pan along with the pam oil for 2 minutes over a low-medium heat. Then, add the entire contents above apart from the dressing and cook for 10-12 minutes stirring frequently. Meanwhile, in a small bowl add the soy sauce, lemon juice, balsamic vinegar, rapeseed oil, salsa and crushed garlic cloves and mix well. When the bean mix is ready add the dressing, and stir through, heat for 2 more minutes, then turn off and leave to stand for 1 minute. Stir through once again and serve immediately.

Nutrition value:

Protein – 36.5g / 12.2g per serving

Carbohydrates – 77.8g / 25.9g per serving

Fat – 18.8g / 6.3g per serving

Total Kcals – 626.4 Kcals / 208.8 Kcals per serving

28. Sweet Chicken Tikka Tortillas
Ingredients:

- 2 white tortillas
- 100g chicken fillet (skinless / chopped)
- 1 handful baby spinach
- 1 medium tomato (chopped into small chunks)
- ¼ cucumber (chopped into small chunks)
- 4 sprays 1 calorie pam oil

- 1 tsp tikka masala seasoning
- ¼ of a lemons juice
- 2 tbsp. natural yogurt
- ½ small red onion (diced)
- 1 tsp fresh mint

Preparation method:

Start by pre-heating a large frying pan with the pam oil over a low-medium heat for 2 minutes. Meanwhile, in a small bowl season the chicken by using your hands to rub the tikka masala evenly all over it and then add the chicken to the pan – cook for 10-12 minutes or until cooked through. Then add the tomato, lemons juice, fresh mint and red onion and cook for a further 6-7 minutes stirring frequently. The final step is to turn the heat off and add the baby spinach, cucumber and natural yogurt, stir the mix well and leave to stand for 1 minute. Put your tortillas in the microwave on full power for 30-40 seconds, put them on a large serving plate add the chicken tikka mix, wrap and enjoy!

Nutrition value

Protein – 37.3g

Carbohydrates – 29.4g

Fat – 4.3g

Total Kcals – 305.5 Kcals

29. Sweet Tuna Salad
Ingredients:

- 1 small tin tuna (60g in water)
- 1 large cherry tomato (chopped into chunks)
- 1 pinch sea salt and black cracked pepper
- 1 sprig rosemary
- 1 tbsp. balsamic vinegar
- 1 tsp olive oil
- 1 tsp lime juice
- 1 tsp lemon juice
- 1 handful baby leaf spinach
- 1 tsp oregano seasoning
- 1 tsp basil seasoning
- ¼ cup chopped cucumber
- 2 spring onions (chopped finely)
- 2 medium celery sticks (chopped)
- ½ green pepper (chopped)

Preparation method:

Pre-heat the oven to 180 degrees. In an oven tray, put down some foil and add the tomato, season with salt and pepper, drizzle with the olive oil and balsamic vinegar, add a rosemary sprig on top and add to the oven for 30 minutes. Once they're ready, heat a frying pan over a low heat and add them along with the rest of the ingredients. Mix well and lightly fry for 67 minutes – stirring frequently.

Nutrition value

Protein – 20g

Carbohydrates – 15.8g

Fat – 15.1g

Total Kcals – 279.1 Kcals

30. Bass Fish Fillet with Fries
Ingredients:

- 100g bass fish fillet
- 100g mixed vegetables (frozen)
- 150g sweet potato (medium sized / skin on, chopped into fries)

- 1 tbsp. rapeseed oil
- ½ tsp parsley
- 1 tsp garlic seasoning
- 1 tsp rosemary seasoning
- 1 tsp sea salt and black cracked pepper
- ½ lemon (chopped into slices)

Preparation method:

Pre-heat your oven to 220 degrees. Start by seasoning the potato fries with the salt and pepper, garlic and rosemary seasoning and drizzle over the rapeseed oil – mix together with your hands evenly. Pre-cook your fries in your microwave on full power for 10 minutes, while you're waiting, it's time to prep your fish. Place a large sheet of foil on the surface, put the fish fillet in the middle and season it with the parsley and place the lemon slices across its length – wrap the fish into a parcel so that all the aroma and flavour stays within and put to one side. Once the fries are pre-cooked, add them along with the fish into the oven for 20-25 mins, occasionally stirring the fries. For the final 10 minutes, add the frozen mixed vegetables to a small pan along with cold water and cook on a medium heat until the boil.

Nutrition value

Protein – 22.5g

Carbohydrates – 34.6g

Fat – 15.1g

Total Kcals – 364.3 Kcals

31. Turkey Burger
Ingredients:

- 100g turkey fillet
- ½ red tomato (sliced)
- 1 wholemeal burger bun
- 1 tbsp. rapeseed oil
- 2 garlic cloves (crushed)
- ½ white onion (finely sliced)
- 1 handful lettuce

Dressing

- 1 tbsp. low fat mayonnaise
- 1 tsp. lime juice
- 1 tsp coriander seasoning
- ½ tsp jerk seasoning

Preparation method:

Pre-heat a large frying pan with the rapeseed oil over a low to medium heat for 2 minutes before adding the white onion and crushed garlic – cook until the onions turn translucent. Then add the turkey fillet and cook for 8-10 minutes turning occasionally, meanwhile, it's time to prepare the dressing. In a small bowl add the mayonnaise, lime juice, coriander, jerk seasoning and use a fork to mix well. Once the turkey fillet is cooked through, empty the contents onto a serving plate, slice the burger bun in half and place it cut side down on the pan for 3-4 mins to lightly toast. Turn the heat off, add the turkey fillet to the bun along with the onions, tomato slices, the pre-made dressing, the lettuce and enjoy!

Nutrition value

Protein – 39.6g

Carbohydrates – 42g

Fat – 20.1g

Total Kcals – 500 Kcals

32. Mixed Beans on Toast

Ingredients:

- 1 wholegrain slice of bread
- 100g reduced salt & sugar baked beans
- 100g mixed beans (in water)
- 1 tsp jerk seasoning

Preparation method:

This is a simple recipe that tastes great and gives an intense energy boost!

Remember before you consume any beans you should always soak them for at least an hour and wash thoroughly to avoid any stomach discomfort and bloating. Wash the mixed beans thoroughly and add them to a small pan along with the baked beans and jerk seasoning. Put the pan over a low heat and simmer for 6-7 minutes – stirring frequently. Then, simply toast the bread and pour the beans on top. Delicious and nutritious!

Nutrition value

Protein – 16.7g

Carbohydrates – 36g

Fat – 2.7g

Total Kcals – 235.1 Kcals

33. Hearty Breakfast

Ingredients:

- 1 wholegrain slice bread
- ½ an avocado (medium, ripened)
- 1 small tomato (quartered)
- 1 tbsp. balsamic vinegar
- 1 pinch sea salt
- ½ tsp oregano seasoning
- 2 large eggs (boiled)
- 1 granny smith apple

Preparation method:

This next recipe is an awesome way to kick start your day, full of nutrients, high in protein, healthy fats and complex carbohydrates to boost your energy levels.

Start by adding 2 eggs to a small pan along with boiling water to cover, boil them over a medium-high heat for 7 minutes then add them to cold water for 2 minutes to cool. Remove them from water and then crack the egg shell several times and leave them to one side for 2-3 minutes – this will make the peeling process easier. Once you've peeled the eggs, cut them both in half and add them to a large serving plate. Toast the bread and then spread with the avocado. Then, quarter the tomato, season with salt, oregano and drizzle with balsamic vinegar. Have with a granny smith apple and enjoy.

Nutrition value

Protein – 22.2g

Carbohydrates – 38.3g

Fat – 24.1g

Total Kcals – 458.9 Kcals

34. Turkey, Rice & Veg (servings: 2)
Ingredients:

- 100g turkey fillet (chopped into chunks)
- 4 sprays 1 calorie pam oil
- 150g wholegrain rice (½ cup uncooked)

- 300ml water
- ¼ cup broccoli (chopped)
- ¼ cup courgette (chopped)
- 1 small tomato (chopped into quarters)
- 50g organic salsa
- 1 tsp jerk seasoning

Preparation method:

Another simple yet delicious and nutritious recipe that is very high in protein, complex carbohydrates and relatively fat free.

Add the rice and 300ml boiling water to a medium sized pan and boil over a medium heat for 12-13 minutes or until all water has been absorbed – stirring frequently. Meanwhile, pre-heat a frying pan along with the pam oil over a low-medium heat for 2 minutes. Season the turkey chunks with the jerk and then add them to the pan – cook for 8-10 minutes or until cooked through. Then, add the broccoli and courgette and cook for a further 3-4 minutes. Add the entire contents to a large serving plate along with the salsa to taste.

Nutrition value:

Protein – 40.9g / 20.4g per serving

Carbohydrates – 56.4g / 28.2g per serving

Fat – 2.1g / 1g per serving

Total Kcals – 408.1 Kcals / 204 Kcals per serving

35. Peanut Butter & Chocolate Sandwich with Banana (servings: 2)

Ingredients:

- 2 slices wholegrain bread
- 1 tbsp. organic peanut butter
- 1 tbsp. chocolate Nutella (or alternative)
- 1 large banana (sliced)

Preparation method:

This next recipe is packed with flavour, great as a snack or desert to cure your cravings that is also high in protein, complex carbohydrates and healthy fats.

Simply spread 1 tbsp. peanut butter on 1 slice of bread and 1 tbsp. Nutella or alternative on the other slice and add the sliced banana in between. Then, add to a George Foreman grill or sandwich toaster and toast until the outside of the bread turns golden brown. Beautiful.

Nutrition value:

Protein – 13.4g / 6.7g per serving

Carbohydrates – 63.3g / 31.6 per serving

Fat – 18g / 9g per serving

Total Kcals – 464.8 Kcals / 232.4 Kcals

36. Bagel with a Treat
Ingredients:

- ½ wholegrain bagel
- 1 tbsp. low fat cheese spread
- 100g Greek yogurt, fat free
- ¼ cup blueberries
- 1 tsp honey

Preparation method:

Simply slice the bagel in half and toast until golden brown and spread with 1 tbsp. low fat cheese. On a side plate add the blueberries, cover with the Greek yogurt and drizzle with honey. Delicious and nutritious!

Nutrition value

Protein – 13.3g

Carbohydrates – 35g

Fat – 6.1g

Total Kcals – 248.1 Kcals

37. Chick Pea Salad (servings: 2)
Ingredients:

- 200g chick peas (tinned in water)
- 6 sprays 1 calorie pam oil
- 1 pinch sea salt & cracked black pepper
- ½ avocado (ripened)
- red pepper (chopped)
- 2 handfuls baby spinach
- 3 garlic cloves (unpeeled)
- ¼ cup cucumber (chopped into small chunks)
- ¼ cup sugar snap peas (chopped)

Dressing

- 1 tbsp. balsamic vinegar
- 1 tsp lemon juice
- 1 tsp sea salt & cracked black pepper

Preparation method:

Again, the first thing you must do to avoid any stomach discomfort and bloating is to leave the peas to soak for at least an hour and then wash thoroughly. Then pre-heat your oven to 180 degrees, grab a large sheet of foil and add the garlic cloves, sprinkle with a pinch of salt and pepper along with 3 sprays of pam oil and make into a tight parcel. Place it in the centre of the oven for 40 minutes or until soft. For the final 10 minutes of the cooking process, preheat a large wok or frying pan along with 3 sprays pam oil over a low heat for 2 minutes before adding the chick peas, red pepper and sugar snap peas – cook for 7-8 minutes stirring frequently. Then, turn the heat off, mash the chick peas up a little with the back end of a spoon, and add the garlic from the oven to the mix – mash and stir again. Finally, add the avocado, baby spinach, cucumber, balsamic vinegar, lemon juice and tsp of sea salt & cracked black pepper – stir well and serve immediately.

Nutrition value:

Protein – 15.8g / 7.9g per serving

Carbohydrates – 65.7g / 32.8g per serving

Fat – 10g / 5g per serving

Total Kcals – 416 Kcals / 208 Kcals per serving

38. Posh Fish & Chips (servings: 2)
Ingredients:

- 200g white potato (medium sized)
- 100g salmon fillet (seasoned with a pinch of sea salt & black pepper)
- 1 tsp rosemary seasoning
- 1 pinch sea salt and black cracked pepper
- 6 sprays 1 calories pam oil
- ½ cup garden peas (frozen)

Preparation method:

Pre-heat your oven to 220 degrees. Peel the potatoes, chop into fries, season with a pinch salt and pepper, 1 tsp rosemary along with 3 sprays 1 calorie pam oil – mix well with your hands. Put them in the microwave for 10 minutes on full power and then put them in the oven for a further 20 minutes. As soon as you place the fries in the oven, pre-heat a medium frying pan over a low-medium heat for 2 minutes before adding the salmon – cook for 18 minutes or until cooked through. For the final 10 minutes of the cooking process, add the frozen peas to a pan along with some cold water to cover, cook over a medium heat until the boil.

Nutrition value:

Protein – 38.2g / 19.1g per serving

Carbohydrates – 59.2g / 29.6g per serving

Fat – 9.9g / 4.9g per serving

Total Kcals – 500 Kcals / 250 Kcals per serving

39. Bed of Avocado + Chocolate Milk (servings: 2)

Ingredients:

- 1 medium avocado (ripened)
- 6-inch granary baguette, cut in half
- 2 pinches sea salt and black cracked pepper
- 1 medium tomato (sliced)
- 400ml chocolate soy milk

Preparation method:

This recipe is simple, great as a snack, high in protein, complex carbohydrates and healthy fats. It's great as an energy booster and to cure cravings.

Simply slice the baguette in half, spread the avocado over both sides, top with the sliced tomato and season with 2 pinches of sea salt & black cracked pepper. Serve with the chocolate soy milk and enjoy!

Nutrition value:

Protein – 23.4g / 11.7g per serving

Carbohydrates – 62.8g / 31.4g per serving

Fat – 21.3g / 10.6g per serving

Total Kcals – 500 Kcals / 250 Kcals per serving

40. Sweet Chicken Curry (servings: 2)

Ingredients:

- 150g 2 minute Palau rice (½ cup / uncle bens)
- 100g chicken fillet (skinless / chopped)
- 1 tbsp. low fat yogurt
- 1 chicken stock cube
- 450ml water (for stock)
- 1 pinch sea salt and cracked black pepper
- ½ tin tomatoes
- 4 sprays 1 calorie pam oil
- 1 tsp coriander seasoning
- ½ white onion (diced)
- 2 garlic cloves (crushed)
- ¼ of a lemons juice
- ¼ of a limes juice
- 1 tbsp. garam-masala seasoning

Preparation method:

Pre-heat a frying pan along with the pam oil over a medium heat for 2 minutes before adding the onion and garlic – cook until the onion turns translucent. Then, add the chopped chicken and cook for 10-12 minutes or until golden brown. Meanwhile, prepare the stock by adding the stock cube along with the 450ml boiling water, coriander and garam-masala to a jug and mix well. Turn the heat down low-medium and add the tinned tomatoes to the pan along with the lemon and limes juice, sea salt and cracked pepper – cook for 3-4 minutes before adding the stock. (add a little stock at a time just covering the mix). Bring to the boil and then turn the heat down low and simmer until the curry mix thickens to your desire. Once the sauce is ready, add the yogurt and mix well – leave to stand for 1 minute and then stir once again. The final step is to simply heat the Palau rice according to packaging and serve to the side of the chicken curry. Your welcome!!

Nutrition value:

Protein – 41.6g / 20.8g per serving

Carbohydrates – 63.6g / 31.8g per serving

Fat – 9.2g / 4.6g per serving

Total Kcals – 500 Kcals / 250 Kcals per serving

41. Chicken Salad with Personality (servings: 2)

Ingredients:

- 100g chicken fillet (skinless / chopped)
- 1 tbsp. jerk seasoning
- 1 tbsp. croutons
- 1 medium tomato (sliced)
- ½ cup cucumber (chopped)
- ½ red onion (sliced thin)
- 1 handful baby leaf spinach
- ½ red pepper (chopped)
- ¼ cup carrot (grated)

Dressing

- 1 tbsp. natural yogurt
- 1 tbsp. balsamic vinegar
- 1 tbsp. rapeseed oil
- 1 tsp lime juice

- 1 tsp lemon juice
- ½ tsp garlic seasoning

Preparation method:

Season the chopped chicken with the jerk and garlic seasoning and put to one side. Pre-heat a large frying pan along with the rapeseed oil for 2 minutes over a medium heat, then add the chicken and cook for 10-12 minutes or until cooked through. The next step is to add the tomato slices, cucumber, red onion, red pepper and cook for a further 4-5 minutes. Then, turn the heat off and add the croutons, baby spinach, grated carrot, natural yogurt and balsamic vinegar – mix together well and eat immediately!

Nutrition value

Protein – 38.7g / 19.3g per serving

Carbohydrates – 42.1g / 21.1g per serving

Fat – 18.8g / 9.4g per serving

Total Kcals – 492.4 Kcals / 246.2 Kcals per serving

42. Banana & Peanut Butter English Muffin with Sweets (servings: 2)

Ingredients:

- 1 wholegrain English muffin
- 1 heaped tbsp. organic peanut butter
- 1 large banana
- ½ cup fresh blueberries

Preparation method:

Once again, another quick and easy recipe that is packed with protein and complex carbohydrates along with some healthy fats. This is a great snack packed with energy to kick start your day.

Simply slice the muffin in half and toast until golden brown and then spread the peanut butter on both slices and then place the sliced bananas on top. Serve them on a medium plate along with the blueberries and enjoy!

Nutrition value:

Protein – 17g / 8.5g per serving

Carbohydrates – 79.2g / 39.6g per serving

Fat – 13.4g / 6.7g per serving

Total Kcals – 500 Kcals / 250 Kcals

43. Chicken Pasta with Greens (servings: 2)

Ingredients:

- 100g chicken fillet (skinless / cut into chunks)
- 3 sprays 1 calorie pam oil
- 150g whole wheat pasta (any style)
- 300ml water
- 100g broccoli (chopped)
- ¼ cup courgette (chopped)
- ½ tin tomatoes
- pinch sea salt and cracked black pepper
- 1 tsp oregano seasoning
- 2 garlic cloves (crushed)
- ½ white onion (finely sliced)
- ¼ of a limes juice

Preparation method:

Pre-heat the frying pan over a medium heat for 2 minutes before adding the pam oil along with the chicken fillet chunks, crushed garlic and diced onion – cook for

10-12 minutes or until cooked through. Then add the pasta to a small pan along with 300ml of cold water, boil over a medium heat on the hob for 10 minutes or until all water has been absorbed. As soon as you've put the pasta on, it's time to prepare the pasta sauce. In the saucepan with the chicken add the tinned tomatoes, salt, pepper, oregano and limes juice along with the courgette and broccoli and lightly simmer until the sauce thickens – stirring frequently. Once the pasta has absorbed all water, simply add to the sauce and mix well. Leave to stand for 1 minute, stir once again and eat immediately!!

Nutrition value:

Protein – 45.6g / 22.8g per serving

Carbohydrates – 61.6g / 30.8g per serving

Fat – 2g / 1g per serving

Total Kcals – 446.8 Kcals / 223.4 Kcals per serving

44. Banana & Blueberry Pancakes (servings: 2)

Ingredients:

- 2 large eggs
- 3 sprays 1 calorie pam oil
- 1 large banana
- ¼ cup blueberries
- 2 tbsp. low fat natural yogurt
- 1 tsp honey

Preparation method:

This recipe is quick and easy and can be enjoyed as a desert or snack at any time of day as part as a healthy diet to cure sweet cravings. Packed with protein, complex carbohydrates and healthy fats to help boost energy levels.

Pre-heat a medium frying pan for 2 minutes over a low-medium heat before adding the pam oil. Then, crush 1 large banana with the back of a fork until you get a slush consistency and put to one side. Next, add 2 eggs to a mixing bowl and mix well before adding the mashed banana and mix together well for 2-3 minutes. Then, crush the fresh blueberries slightly with the back of a fork and add to the egg and banana mix and mix well again. Once the pancake batter is ready use a ladle or scooper to scoop out some of the mix one scoop at a time and place it in the middle of the pan gently. Leave for 60-90 seconds before flipping over and then repeat the process. Absolutely scrumptious!!

Nutrition method

Protein – 20.6g / 10.3g per serving

Carbohydrates – 55.5g / 27.7g per serving

Fat – 18.1g / 9g per serving

Total Kcals – 467.3 Kcals / 233.6 Kcals per serving

45. Creamy Tuna Pasta (servings: 2)
Ingredients:

- 150g whole wheat penne (uncooked)
- 300ml water
- 1 small tin tuna (60g in water)
- ½ tin tomatoes

- 1 tbsp. rapeseed oil
- 1 tsp oregano seasoning
- 1 tsp cayenne pepper
- 1 pinch sea salt and cracked black pepper
- 2 cloves garlic (crushed)
- ½ a limes juice
- 1 tbsp. low fat natural yogurt
- 15g parmesan cheese (grated)

Preparation method:

Add the penne to a medium pan along with the 300ml water and boil for 10 minutes or until all water has been absorbed. While you're waiting, pre-heat a frying pan for 2 minutes over a low-medium heat before adding the rapeseed oil and tuna – cook for 2-3 minutes stirring frequently. Then, add the tinned tomatoes along with the lime juice, crushed garlic, oregano seasoning, cayenne seasoning and salt & pepper seasoning. Simmer for 10 minutes or until the sauce thickens. Once the pasta is ready add it to the sauce, turn the heat off, mix well and add the parmesan cheese – mix lightly and leave for 1 minute. Finally, add the tablespoon of low fat yogurt and stir through the mix well. Simply delicious.

Nutrition value

Protein – 29.8g / 14.9g per serving

Carbohydrate – 47.8g / 23.9g per serving

Fat – 18.2g / 9.1g per serving

Total Kcals – 474.2 Kcals / 237.1 Kcals per serving

46. Sticky Jerk Chicken (servings: 2)
Ingredients:

- 100g chicken fillet (skinless)
- ½ red pepper (chopped)
- 3 sticks of asparagus (chopped)
- 100g broccoli (chopped)
- 3 sprays 1 calorie pam oil
- 1 pinch sea salt and black cracked pepper

Sauce

- 1 tsp jerk
- 3 tbsp. soy sauce

- 1 tbsp. rapeseed oil
- 2 garlic cloves (crushed)
- 1 tsp ginger seasoning
- ½ tsp chilli flakes
- ¼ of a limes juice
- 1 pinch sea salt and black cracked pepper
- 1 tsp honey

Preparation method:

For best results, it is best to marinate the chicken over night or for at least a few hours. In a large serving bowl add all ingredients above for the sauce to the chicken fillet – using your hands, mix well, cover with foil and store in the fridge to marinate. Once you've done that, simply add the chicken mix to your oven – cook for 25-30 minutes at 200 degrees. For the final 10 minutes of the cooking process, pre-heat your frying pan over a low-medium heat for 2 minutes before adding the pam oil along with the broccoli, asparagus and red pepper – season with salt & pepper and lightly fry.

Nutrition value

Protein – 41.5g / 20.7g per serving

Carbohydrates – 32.7g / 16.3g per serving

Fat – 14g / 7g per serving

Total Kcals – 422.8 Kcals / 211.4 Kcals per serving

47. Fruit & Berry Porridge (servings: 2)
Ingredients:

- ¼ cup oats
- ¼ cup water
- ½ cup soya milk (unsweetened)
- 1 tsp Nutella chocolate (or alternative)
- 1 tsp cinnamon
- ¼ cup dried mixed berries
- 1 small apple (peeled & chopped into small chunks)

Preparation method:

Simple, quick and easy, nutritious recipe to kick start your day and boost your energy levels.

Add the oats along with the water, soya milk, cinnamon, mixed berries and apple chunks to a pan and put on the hob over a low heat for 6-7 minutes or until the porridge thickens to your desire – stirring frequently. Then, empty the contents into a large serving bowl and add the Nutella into the centre of the porridge and leave to stand for 1 minute. Stir well and eat immediately!

Nutrition value

Protein – 9.6g / 4.8 per serving

Carbohydrates – 68.2g / 34.1g per serving

Fat – 12g / 6g per serving

Total Kcals – 419.2 Kcals / 209.6 Kcals per serving

48. Egg & Bacon English Muffin
Ingredients:

- 1 wholegrain English muffin
- 2 slices lean bacon (cut any excess fat off)

- 3 sprays 1 calorie pam oil
- 1 large egg
- 1 tbsp. low fat butter
- 1 tbsp. reduced salt and sugar ketchup

Preparation method:

To begin with, add 1 egg to a small pan along with boiling water to cover. Boil the egg over a medium-high heat on the hob for 7 minutes, then drain and add cold water – leave to cool for 1 minute before draining. Crack the egg several times with a fork and leave for 2 minutes then peel it, cut in half and leave to one side. Then, pre-heat a frying pan on the hob over a low-medium heat before adding the pam oil along with the 2 slices of lean bacon – cook for 8-10 minutes or until crisp. Finally, slice the English muffin in half, toast, spread butter on both halves and add the bacon, egg and red sauce between the two slices and enjoy!

Nutrition value

Protein – 33g

Carbohydrates – 40.5g

Fat – 17.3g

Total Kcals – 449.7 Kcals

49. Jamaican Inspired Rice & Peas – simmer 60 mins (servings: 3)

Ingredients:

- 2 garlic cloves (crushed)
- 1 medium white onion (thinly sliced)
- 1 tsp jerk seasoning
- 1 tsp Cajun seasoning
- ½ a limes juice
- 2 medium spring onions (chopped into small pieces)
- 1 sprig of fresh thyme
- 1 pinch sea salt and black pepper
- ½ cup coconut milk (unsweetened)
- 150g wholegrain rice (½ cup)
- 300ml water (for rice)
- 1 tsp hot cayenne pepper
- 100g garden peas (frozen)

- 100g red kidney beans (tinned in water)

Preparation method:

This next recipe has a lot of ingredients that'll leave your taste buds tingling, it's very simple it just takes a little time to allow all the flavours to combine together, to create the perfect aroma.

Start by washing the red kidney beans thoroughly and then simply add the entire ingredients above in a large pot pan and put on the hob over a low heat and simmer for 1 hour or until the mix thickens to your desire – stir occasionally.

Nutrition value

Protein – 19g / 6.3g per serving

Carbohydrates – 87.5g / 29.2g per serving

Fat – 6.4g / 2.1g per serving

Total Kcals – 483.6 Kcals / 161.2 Kcals per serving

50. Chicken Fried Rice (servings: 2)

Ingredients:

- 1 chicken fillet (100g skinless & chopped)
- 150g white rice (½ cup)
- 2 spring onions (diced)
- ½ large white onion (diced)
- 2 garlic cloves (crushed)
- 4 sprays 1 calorie pam oil
- ¼ cup garden peas (tinned in water)
- ¼ cup carrots (diced)
- 1 pinch sea salt and cracked black pepper
- ½ tsp ginger seasoning

Preparation method:

For best results and to get the perfect texture to this dish, pre-make the rice and store in the fridge for 60 minutes before adding to the pan. To do this, simply add the rice along with 300ml boiling water to a medium pan and boil over a medium heat on the hob for 10-12 minutes or until all water has been absorbed – store in the fridge for 1 hour. Once you've prepared the rice, it's time for the next stage. Pre-heat a frying over a low-medium heat on the hob for 2 minutes before adding the pam oil, garlic and white onion – cook until the onion turns translucent. Then, add the chopped chicken and cook until golden brown. Next, turn the heat down low and add the spring onions, garden peas, carrots, salt, black pepper and ginger seasoning to the pan – cook for 6-7 minutes before adding the rice (stirring frequently). Cook for a further 3-4 minutes stirring occasionally and then serve immediately!

Nutrition value:

Protein – 42.5g / 21.2g per serving

Carbohydrates – 71.2g / 35.6g per serving

Fat – 4.4g / 2.2g per serving

Total Kcals – 494.4 Kcals / 247.2 Kcals per serving

Conclusion

Thank you again for purchasing this book on the best way to implement a Low Carb Diet in your eating program!

I hope this book was able to help you to gain insights about the principles of a low carb diet and the strategies that you can use to achieve the body that you have been dreaming of.

The next step is to get started!

The tips in this book won't give you drastic results. What you have been given are flexible and doable strategies to get you started on a low carb diet. Putting these strategies to practice is up to you. How dedicated you are with your diet strategies will determine your success. The low carb diet works, but only if you stick to what it requires.

Once you are comfortable with the lenient and easy to follow low carb strategy described in this book, you can move on to more restrictive diets if you wish to achieve faster results. The important thing is to condition your body to a low carb diet or at least a semi-restricted carb diet. Once you have taken that first step, you can move on to further weight loss using more stringent low carb diet solutions.

About The Author

Francis Sherman loves low carb cooking The author has written several recipe books on the topic. He has served as an instructor promoting various cusine arts in indie shows and fairs. He is currently living with his spouse in Texas.

www.ingramcontent.com/pod-product-compliance
Lightning Source LLC
LaVergne TN
LVHW011945070526
838202LV00054B/4803